Patricia Danell

MANIFESTING REALITY: DOLORES CANNON'S JOURNEY THROUGH TIME AND CONSCIOUSNESS

Patricia Danell

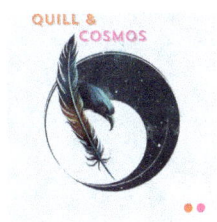

Patricia Danell

Copyright © 2024 Patricia Danell

All rights reserved

DEDICATION

To you, the reader and traveler of this extraordinary journey,

This book is dedicated to all those who dared to dream and had the courage to believe that those dreams could become reality. It is for the explorers of the unknown, the builders of worlds, and the daydreamers who see beyond the visible and touch the invisible with the strength of their spirit.

To you, who have never given up on the quest for a fuller, richer, and more authentic life. May these pages serve as a guide and inspiration along the path to your highest realization and the discovery of your true power.

And finally, to Dolores Cannon, whose wisdom and teachings have illuminated this path. May her legacy continue to inspire generations of spiritual seekers, encouraging them to look deeper within and further out.

With love and light, this book comes to life, hoping to ignite a spark in the depths of your being and accompany you in the magnificent art of creating your reality.

Patricia Danell

TABLE OF CONTENTS

1	BRIEF BIOGRAPHY OF DOLORES CANNON	N. pag.9
2	OVERVIEW OF THE CONCEPT OF MANIFESTATION	N. pag.13
3	THE IMPORTANCE OF AWARENESS AND INTENTION IN CREATING REALITY	N. pag.23
4	FOUNDATIONS OF QUANTUM REALITY	N. pag.32
5	HOW QUANTUM PHYSICS APPLIES TO MANIFESTATION	N. pag.43
6	THE MIND-UNIVERSE CONNECTION	N. pag.51
7	PRINCIPLES OF SYNCHRONICITY AND CONNECTION	N. pag.60
8	LESSONS FROM DOLORES CANNON	N. pag.65
9	SUMMARY OF DOLORES CANNON'S MOST INFLUENTIAL DISCOVERIES	N. pag.74
10	APPLICATION OF D. CANNON'S TECHNIQUES IN EVERYDAY LIFE	N. pag.77
11	PREPARATION FOR MANIFESTATION	N. pag.81
12	TECHNIQUES FOR CLARIFYING AND PURIFYING INTENTIONS	N. pag.87
13	MEDITATION AND VISUALIZATION: OTHER GUIDED PRACTICES TO ESTABLISH A DEEP CONNECTION WITH INTENTION	N. pag.99
14	ADDRESSING AND RELEASING	N. pag.103

ENERGY BLOCKS

15	TOOLS AND TECHNIQUES FOR MANIFESTATION	N. pag.106
16	CREATING A DAILY ROUTINE	N. pag.112
17	JOURNALING AND PROGRESS TRACKING	N. pag.115
18	STORIES OF SUCCESS	N. pag.122
19	ANALYSIS OF WHAT WORKED AND WHAT DIDN'T	N. pag.128
20	OVERCOMING CHALLENGES	N. pag.136
21	MAINTAINING MOTIVATION	N. pag.144
22	ADAPTABILITY AND RESILIENCE	N. pag.150
23	CONCLUSION	N. pag.155
24	CALL TO ACTION	N. pag.158
25	FINAL REFLECTIONS	N. pag.162
26	APPENDIX: ADDITIONAL RESOURCES	N. pag.167
27	GLOSSARY	N. pag.172

BRIEF BIOGRAPHY OF DOLORES CANNON

INTRODUCTION TO HER BACKGROUND AND HER MAJOR WORKS

Dolores Cannon (1931-2014) was an American hypnotherapist and writer, whose work explored the boundaries between science, spirituality, and unexplained phenomena. Her career spanned almost five decades during which she developed and perfected a hypnosis technique she herself called Quantum Healing Hypnosis Technique (QHHT), a methodology that allows access to past lives and the Higher Self for healing and introspection purposes.

Born in Missouri, Cannon began her career as a hypnotherapist in the 1960s, initially working with her husband in a hypnosis practice for weight loss and smoking cessation. At the start of her career, Dolores Cannon primarily focused on hypnosis for weight control and smoking cessation. However, a crucial event during a routine hypnosis session marked a decisive turning point in her professional and scientific journey. During a session in the 1960s, while working with a client for a common health issue, the subject unexpectedly entered a much deeper trance state than usual.

In this trance state, the client began speaking with a voice and tone that were not their usual, describing experiences that could not be attributed to their current life. They began providing vivid and coherent details of past existences, shifting from one era to another and from one geography to another with extraordinary precision. These narratives were not only detailed but also included specific cultural and historical elements that were difficult to explain without prior knowledge of the topics discussed.

Initially skeptical, Dolores was struck by the wealth of information and the naturalness with which the client described these supposed past lives. What made these episodes even more intriguing was that the client, once back in a normal state of consciousness, had no recollection of the information they provided during the trance.

This incident prompted deep reflection and a radical change in Dolores's approach to hypnosis practice. She realized that what she had observed could extend well beyond the traditional applications of hypnosis. Intrigued by the potential of this discovery and driven by growing curiosity, Dolores began systematically studying and documenting other similar cases. This led her to develop a new field of interest and specialize in past-life regression, delving into specific techniques to facilitate and study these experiences.

The decision to explore this new territory not only enriched her professional practice but also paved the way for what would become the centerpiece of her future career: the use of past-life regression for therapeutic and exploration purposes of the human consciousness. Over time, this approach became a distinctive feature of her work, contributing to shaping the foundation of her theories and subsequent publications.

Dolores published her first book, "Five Lives Remembered," in 1980, followed by "Jesus and the Essenes" and "Between Death and Life," the latter being a detailed exploration of the afterlife experience as reported by her clients during hypnosis sessions. These works laid the groundwork for her reputation as one of the most innovative figures in the field of past-life regression.

Perhaps the best-known among her works is the series "The Convoluted Universe," which began in 2001. This series, comprising five volumes, explores themes such as reincarnation, aliens, lives on other planets and dimensions, as well as the physical and spiritual laws governing the universe. These books reflect the breadth of Dolores's interests and the depth of her research, taking readers on a journey through the mysterious and the occult with a clear and engaging narrative approach.

Dolores Cannon has left a lasting legacy through her books, seminars, and QHHT, significantly contributing to the understanding of the human unconscious and providing tools for personal and spiritual healing. Her ability to narrate complex stories in an accessible manner has made her works essential for anyone interested in exploring the mysteries of life and existence beyond the boundaries of traditional science.

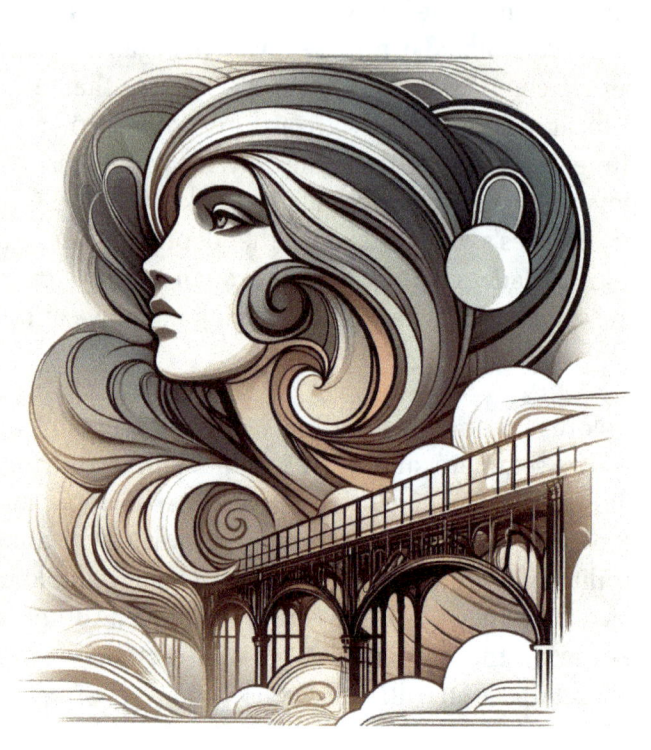

OVERVIEW OF THE CONCEPT OF MANIFESTATION

DEFINITION OF MANIFESTATION AND HOW IT RELATES TO THE TEACHINGS OF D. CANNON

Overview of the Concept of Manifestation

Manifestation, a concept that evokes an echo of limitless possibility, is an intriguing phenomenon situated at the intersection of individual will and the continuum of existence itself. This process is not merely a function of desire or ambition, but a complex and deeply intentional practice of personal and universal realization.

Nature and Mechanisms of Manifestation

At its core, manifestation entails tangibly bringing into being what previously existed only in the realm of thought, emotion, or aspiration. This psyche alchemy transforms dreams (the ineffable) into tangible reality, employing the potent synergy between mind and matter. It is a refined art that requires not only clarity of intent but also a profound synchronization with the subtler laws governing the universe.

The manifestation process operates on two fundamental levels:

1. Internally, through the calibration of our consciousness, which encompasses thoughts, beliefs, emotions, and expectations. These mental and emotional elements must be aligned cohesively and focusedly. Clear intention and positive vision are essential, as they generate a vibrational frequency that can attract similar circumstances.

2. Externally, by interacting with the surrounding environment and the broader universe. This interaction is based on the premise that everything in the universe is interconnected and that every thought or action sends waves through this interconnected field, influencing and altering external reality.

The Role of the Human Mind

At the heart of manifestation lies the extraordinary ability of the human mind to influence and shape its environment. Every thought produces a resonance, a vibration that extends beyond the physical boundaries of the brain, interacting with energy and matter. This ability to send and receive frequencies is what enables individuals to "tune in" to the realities they wish to manifest.

The Principle of Resonance

Fundamental to the manifestation process is the principle of resonance, which states that similar frequencies attract. In the context of manifestation, this means that maintaining an emotional and mental frequency that matches what one wishes to attract is crucial. This tuning is not passive but requires active and conscious participation to cultivate and maintain desired emotional and mental states.

Effective Manifestation Practices

Manifestation requires more than mere desire or positive thinking; it necessitates consistent and intentional practices, such as:

- **Creative Visualization**: Vividly imagining the desired outcome as if it were already accomplished. This establishes a clear and powerful connection with the object of one's desires.

- **Positive Affirmations:** Repeating statements that reinforce the desired reality helps reshape limiting beliefs and align the mind with goals.

- **Meditation and Mindfulness**: These practices help maintain a focused and serene mind, enhancing the ability to stay tuned into desired frequencies without being overwhelmed by doubt or negativity.

Ultimately, manifestation is a continuous dialogue between inner desire and universal energy, a dynamic process that requires understanding, patience, and persistence. It is the art of shaping not only one's own destiny but, in a sense, also the fabric of reality itself. Engaging in this practice is not merely about achieving personal goals but about participating in a grander cosmic play, where each individual's creations contribute to the collective experience.

Basic Theory of Manifestation

According to the principles of quantum physics, every reality is potentially infinite; every choice, thought, or action branches out into an incalculable number of parallel universes. Manifestation harnesses this infinite network of possibilities through the focus of intention. More precisely, it is believed that through the conscious use of thought and emotion — powerful and directional energies in themselves — one can influence which branch of potentiality becomes reality in the material world.

Dolores Cannon and Manifestation

Dolores Cannon, throughout her prolific career, deeply explored the concept of manifestation through her innovative Quantum Healing Hypnosis Technique (QHHT). This technique, which she developed and refined, allows access to very deep trance states during which subjects can explore past lives and establish a direct connection with their Higher Self. Through QHHT, Cannon discovered and compellingly demonstrated how thoughts and intentions are not mere products of the mind but actual agents of change in the fabric of reality.

Depth of QHHT and Manifestation

In her hypnosis sessions, Cannon guided her clients through an inner journey where hidden or dormant information often emerged from the subconscious. These sessions revealed that many of the physical and emotional limitations experienced by individuals were closely linked to their inner beliefs and thought patterns. Dolores repeatedly observed that by changing these patterns, people began to manifest changes not only internally but also externally, such as improvements in health, relationships, and life circumstances.

Interaction between Thought, Emotion, and Physical Reality

According to Cannon, thoughts generate emotions, and together they form a force that can alter physical reality. This concept is rooted in the notion that the subconscious does not differentiate between what is real and what is imagined. When thoughts and emotions are powerful enough, the subconscious interprets them as actual realities, prompting the individual to operate in ways that can manifest these new "realities" in the physical world.

The Role of the Subconscious in Manifestation

Cannon emphasized the crucial role of the subconscious in the manifestation process. She viewed this part of the mind as a bridge between conscious desire and unconscious realization. The subconscious, with its vast ability to influence behavior and almost automatic reactions, can be programmed or reprogrammed through conscious thoughts and focused intentions. During QHHT sessions, Cannon worked to bring these unconscious aspects to the surface, allowing individuals to recognize and restructure limiting patterns and harness this powerful internal resource to actively change their reality.

Practice of Manifestation through QHHT

In practice, through QHHT, clients were guided to intensely visualize and emotionally feel what they desired to manifest. Cannon led them to imagine scenarios where they had already achieved their goals, from achieving physical healing to overcoming personal or professional obstacles. This technique not only helped establish new positive beliefs but also activated a physical and emotional response that aligned the individual with their desires, speeding up the manifestation process.

Dolores Cannon's discoveries and methods offer a profound understanding of how powerful our inner selves can be in shaping the external. Her work underscores that manifestation is not an external or mysterious phenomenon but an accessible and manageable process that begins within us. With the right awareness and techniques, according to Cannon, each of us has the power to transform our lives, realizing manifestations that reflect our deepest desires and aspirations.

Implications and Practical Applications

Dolores Cannon greatly deepened the dynamics of manifestation, providing not only a robust theoretical foundation but also practical tools for her students and readers. In addition to recognizing the fluid and dynamic nature of reality, which continuously responds to our thoughts and emotions, Cannon emphasized how we can actively participate in and influence this process to bring about positive changes in our lives.

Clarification of Intentions

One of the most critical aspects highlighted by Cannon is the clarification of intentions. This process goes beyond mere desire or hope; it requires a precise understanding of what one wishes to achieve. Clarity of intentions involves detailed goal setting, which should be specific, measurable, achievable, relevant, and time-bound (SMART). Cannon advised writing intentions down, deeply reflecting on them, and periodically reviewing them to maintain focus. This helps consolidate the desire in the subconscious, making the manifestation process more effective.

Maintaining a Positive Emotional and Mental State

Cannon placed particular emphasis on the need to cultivate and maintain a positive emotional and mental state. This does not mean ignoring or suppressing negative emotions but rather recognizing, accepting, and transforming them. A positive attitude facilitates a higher vibration, which is essential for attracting desired events, situations, and responses. Positivity generates resilience and openness, necessary elements for overcoming any obstacles or delays in the manifestation process.

Practical Techniques: Visualization, Affirmation, and Meditation

Dolores Cannon taught specific techniques to activate and sustain manifestation:

- **Visualization**: This technique involves creating a vivid mental image of the desired goal, imagining oneself already living that reality. Cannon suggested practicing visualization regularly, preferably in a state of deep relaxation to facilitate impression on the subconscious.

- **Affirmation**: Positive affirmations are statements that reinforce the ability to achieve goals and improve one's mental and emotional state. Cannon recommended repeating these affirmations daily, especially in the morning and evening, to instill empowering beliefs.

- **Meditation**: The practice of meditation helps center and calm the mind, making it more receptive and less disturbed by destructive thoughts or stress. Meditation not only helps maintain clear focus on intentions but also opens the mind to receiving insights and inspirations that can guide further actions toward manifestation.

Broader Implications

Dolores Cannon's work illustrates how reality, far from being a static fact, is a continuously woven fabric of our thoughts and emotions. This concept not only offers a sense of power and agency but also imposes significant responsibility: we are co-creators of our existence and, on a broader level, of the world we inhabit. With the right guidance and understanding of Cannon's techniques, it becomes possible not only to shape one's own destiny but also to positively influence the environment and surrounding communities.

Through the practical application of these teachings, we can not only pursue personal transformation but also contribute to the creation of a collective reality that reflects higher values of awareness, empathy, and collaboration.

Conclusion

In delineating manifestation as both a concept and a practice, Dolores Cannon has left a legacy of empowerment and responsibility. Through her methods, she teaches us that each of us has access to powerful tools to not only navigate but also create our own reality. Manifestation, as interpreted and taught by Cannon, is not just an act of personal creation but a continuous dialogue with the universe, an interaction resonating with the deepest truths of our existence.

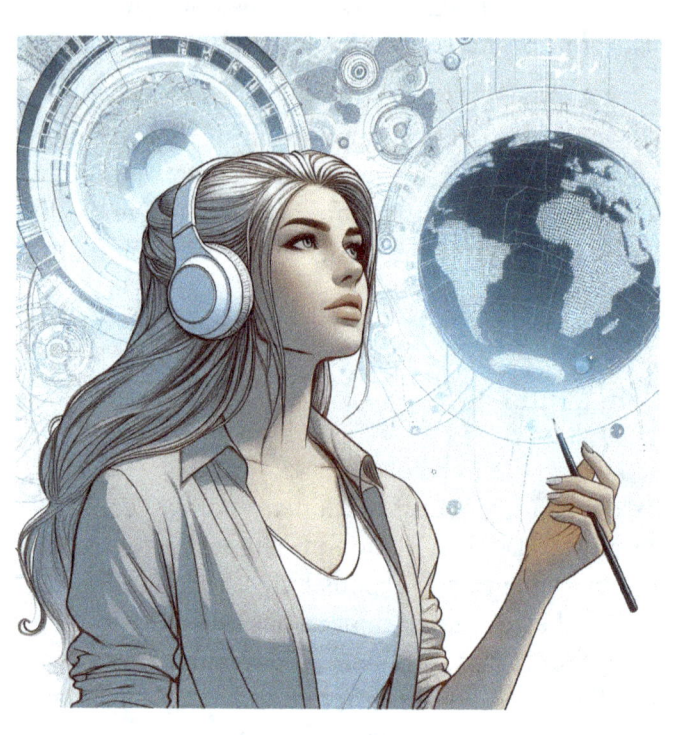

THE IMPORTANCE OF AWARENESS AND INTENTION IN CREATING REALITY

INTRODUCTION TO THE KEY CONCEPTS THAT WILL BE EXPLORED IN THE BOOK

The importance of Awareness and Intention in Reality Creation

Introduction to Key Concepts

The reality we experience each day is not a fixed stage upon which we passively act, but rather a field of infinite possibilities that actively responds to our presence and participation. At the heart of this dynamic interaction between the individual and the universe lie two fundamental concepts: awareness and intention. These elements not only shape our experience of the world but, as suggested by the research and practices of Dolores Cannon, have the power to literally transform the canvas of reality.

Awareness: Gateway to Deep Perception

Awareness is not merely a word describing a generic attention to the present, but represents a deep immersion in the entirety of the human experience. Being aware means fully embracing the current moment, being completely present not only physically but also mentally and emotionally. This implies a keen awareness of oneself, one's environment, and the dynamics that govern every action and reaction.

Beyond the Surface of External Stimuli

Awareness goes far beyond simply responding to external stimuli. It is an active and continuous recognition of the subtle, often invisible forces that shape and profoundly influence our life experience. These forces can be internal, such as our unexpressed thoughts or repressed emotions, or external, such as cultural expectations or social pressures. Awareness of these factors is crucial as it provides the foundation upon which we can build conscious and meaningful intentions.

The Need for a Solid Foundation

Without a foundation of awareness, every attempt at manifestation may result in confusion, disorder, or even counterproductivity. Manifestation requires a solid ground of clarity and understanding, without which intentions can be misdirected or influenced by inauthentic desires. It is awareness that enables us to discern between what is truly desired and what is merely a conditioned reflection of non-authentic needs.

A Process of Self-Exploration

The path to awareness requires a constant and honest examination of what truly animates our being: rooted beliefs, emotions that fluctuate beneath the surface, and thoughts that form the fabric of our daily reality. This process of self-exploration is deep and often requires confronting aspects of oneself that may be uncomfortable or difficult to accept. However, it is only through this sincere introspection that we can hope to free ourselves from the chains of old thought patterns that limit us.

Freedom from Limiting Influences

As awareness grows, one begins to recognize and distance oneself from external influences that may have subtly shaped our perceptions and reactions. This detachment does not imply a withdrawal from the world but a more authentic and conscious participation. It is a process of disidentification from thought patterns that no longer serve us, thus allowing for true personal transformation that manifests in choices and actions that are freer and in line with our true desires.

Awareness as a Foundation for Personal Growth

Ultimately, awareness is not only a necessary component for effective manifestation; it is also an essential practice for personal and spiritual well-being. It enables a richer and fuller existence, in which each moment is lived with intensity and each decision is made with deliberation. With deep awareness, we can not only navigate but also actively shape the reality around us, making choices that reflect our deepest values and highest aspirations.

Intention: The Engine of Manifestation

Intention emerges as the true engine of manifestation, transforming awareness and understanding into concrete actions and tangible results. It goes beyond being a mere wish or a vague goal; it takes the form of a deep and determined commitment, a genuine energetic command sent out to the universe to catalyze change.

Definition and Power of Intention

An effective intention is much more than a passive thought; it is an act of will that synthesizes desire, determination, and direction. It manifests as a clear vision, often accompanied by a specific articulation of what one wishes to achieve. This vision is neither vague nor uncertain but is precisely outlined and committed to. Intentions are like arrows aimed at specific targets; their strength lies in their ability to penetrate obstacles and direct energy toward well-defined goals.

The Precision of Intentions

Clarity is crucial when formulating intentions. A well-defined and detailed intention significantly increases the likelihood of success because it maps out a clear path to follow. For example, instead of having the generic intention of "being happy," a more precise intention could be "finding joy in my daily work by the end of the year." This specifies not only the desired goal but also a timeframe and specific context, which help focus energy more effectively.

Energy and Consistency in Intention

The strength of an intention also stems from the constancy and coherence of the mental and emotional energy invested. It is not enough to simply formulate an intention; it must be nurtured with consistent thoughts, words, and actions. This consistent support creates a vibrational field that is in resonance with the desired goal, facilitating its manifestation in the physical world. Like a magnet attracting metal objects, a powerful intention attracts the necessary circumstances for goal achievement.

Trust and Surrender to the Universe

A crucial component of intention is trust, which must permeate the manifestation process. After clearly formulating the intention and dedicating constant energy to it, it is essential to "release" it into the universe. This does not mean relinquishing control or interest but rather trusting in the belief that the universe will cooperate in achieving the goal. This act of trust eliminates tension and worry that could otherwise sabotage the manifestation process.

Intention thus acts as a potent catalyst in the manifestation process, transforming awareness into action and desires into reality. It is a delicate balance between active determination and trusting surrender, between specificity and openness. Navigating this balance requires practice, patience, and, above all, a deep understanding of oneself and the universal laws that govern manifestation. With the right intention, we can not only aspire to change our lives but actually do so, actively shaping the reality that surrounds us.

Integration of Awareness and Intention

The effective combination of awareness and intention represents a powerful dynamic in the process of manifestation. This synergy not only optimizes the path to achieving personal and spiritual goals but also transforms the way we interact with the world.

Awareness as the Foundation

Awareness acts as the foundation upon which every meaningful intent is built. Being fully aware means having a comprehensive and clear understanding not only of one's internal emotions and thoughts but also of the surrounding environment and interactions taking place. This profound awareness enables the recognition not only of opportunities that arise but also of challenges and obstacles that may arise. With this knowledge, one can navigate through the complexity of their experiences and relationships more confidently, making informed choices that truly reflect their values and aspirations.

Intention as Direction

While awareness provides the map, intention serves as the compass, guiding deliberate and targeted actions toward established goals. A clear and well-defined intention allows for the efficient focus of energies and resources, avoiding distractions and minimizing unnecessary efforts. Intention crystallizes desire into an action plan that can be followed precisely, whether for personal improvements, relational changes, or professional achievements.

Synergy and Practical Application in QHHT

Dolores Cannon perfectly illustrates this synergy through her Quantum Healing Hypnosis Technique (QHHT) method. During a QHHT session, subjects are guided into a state of deep hypnotic awareness, where they can explore and recognize subconscious patterns and limiting beliefs that have hitherto guided, often unconsciously, their decisions and behaviors. With this revelation, subjects gain the ability to review and reformulate their intentions with newfound clarity, directing themselves toward goals that more faithfully reflect their true desires and aspirations.

Transforming Beliefs into Actions

Once these limiting beliefs have been identified and understood, subjects can then establish precise intentions to modify or eliminate them. This process of transforming beliefs into concrete actions is an excellent example of how awareness and intention can work together to create real and lasting changes. The new intentions, supported by a deeper and more authentic understanding of the self, lead to choices and behaviors that are in harmony with one's deepest values.

Tangible Results and Creation of New Realities

The result of this synergy is the ability not only to dream or aspire to a certain reality but to actually create it. Individuals become active co-creators in their lives, using awareness and intention to actively shape their existence. In this way, the manifestation process becomes a journey of personal growth and transformation, where every step is informed and intentional, every choice is powerful, and every result is a direct reflection of personal power.

The importance of awareness and intention in creating reality cannot be underestimated. They are the keys that unlock the doors of human and cosmic potential, allowing individuals to exert a conscious and creative influence on their lives and, by extension, the world around them. By exploring and applying these concepts, we can discover not only how to shape our experiences but also how to actively contribute to the co-creation of a collectively enriched and meaningful existence.

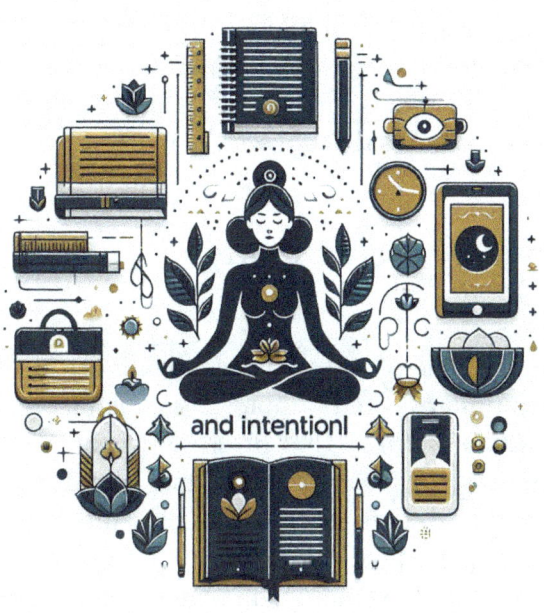

FOUNDATIONS OF QUANTUM REALITY

THEORY OF QUANTUM REALITY

Quantum reality represents one of the most fascinating and challenging fields of study of the twentieth century, continuing to intrigue both collective imagination and scientific inquiry in the twenty-first. At the heart of this theory lies a revolutionary concept: the microscopic world, governed by the laws of quantum mechanics, behaves in ways that defy intuition and the laws of classical physics that govern the macroscopic world.

Wave-Particle Duality

The principle of wave-particle duality is one of the most revolutionary and thought-provoking concepts of quantum physics. This principle states that subatomic particles, such as electrons and photons, can exhibit properties of both discrete particles and extended waves. This apparent contradiction not only challenges our classical understanding of matter and energy but also opens the door to a deeper understanding of the fundamental workings of the universe.

Historical and Experimental Origins

The theory of wave-particle duality was first introduced by Louis de Broglie in the 1920s, a proposal that extended the concept of duality already suggested by research on light. Before de Broglie, light had been described both as a wave (demonstrated by interference experiments) and as a particle (highlighted by the photoelectric effect for which Albert Einstein received the Nobel Prize). De Broglie proposed that this duality was not limited to light but was a universal characteristic of all particles. The double-slit experiment, originally conducted with light and later replicated with electrons, is one of the fundamental experiments demonstrating this duality. When a stream of electrons is fired through two closely spaced slits, instead of forming two distinct groups of impacts on the detection screen, the electrons form an interference pattern reminiscent of that created by water waves. This interference pattern suggests that each electron passes through both slits simultaneously, like a wave, and then interferes with itself.

Philosophical and Practical Implications

Wave-particle duality challenges the classical principle of identity, which asserts that every entity is identical to itself and cannot be something else at the same time. Instead, in quantum mechanics, a particle can also be a wave, depending on how it is measured or observed. This has profound implications for the concept of reality, suggesting that the properties of subatomic particles are somehow dependent on observation, a theme that touches on issues of perception, knowledge, and reality itself. On a practical level, wave-particle duality has significant applications in technologies such as electron microscopy and semiconductor manufacturing. In these fields, exploiting the wave nature of electrons allows scientists and engineers to observe and manipulate structures much smaller than those that could be achieved using only visible light. Wave-particle duality remains one of the most fascinating and counterintuitive concepts in modern physics. It continues to be a subject of intense research, not only to better understand how particles behave at the quantum level but also to explore the theoretical and practical implications of this behavior in fields ranging from quantum cryptography to quantum computing. This principle, therefore, not only alters our understanding of the microscopic world but also prompts us to reconsider the laws we believe govern reality on a larger scale.

Indeterminacy and Superposition

Heisenberg's Uncertainty Principle

Heisenberg's uncertainty principle stands as one of the cornerstones of quantum mechanics, introducing a concept that is as counterintuitive as it is fundamental to understanding nature at the subatomic level. Formulated in 1927 by Werner Heisenberg, the principle states that it is impossible to simultaneously determine both the position and momentum (or velocity) of a particle with absolute precision. More precisely, the attempt to precisely measure one of these variables leads to an inevitable loss of precision in the other. This uncertainty is not due to imperfections in measurement tools or experimental techniques but is an intrinsic property of the quantum nature of things. The uncertainty principle underscores the idea that at the quantum level, reality is not fixed or rigidly determined but is inherently probabilistic. In other words, quantum phenomena cannot be predicted with absolute certainty but only in terms of probabilities.

Quantum Superposition

Extending the concept of uncertainty, quantum superposition pushes the boundaries of our understanding of reality. This principle states that particles, such as electrons or photons, can exist in multiple states simultaneously until they are observed or measured. In practical terms, this means that a particle can be in different locations or have different energy states simultaneously, and only the act of observation "decides" the particle's definitive state.

This concept is vividly illustrated by Schrödinger's cat thought experiment. In this scenario, a cat is placed in a sealed box with a mechanism that can release poison based on the radioactive decay of an atom, an event subject to the laws of quantum mechanics. Until the box is opened, the atom must be considered both decayed and not decayed, so the cat must be considered both alive and dead, existing in a superposition of states. Only by opening the box, observing the system, does this superposition collapse into a defined state.

Implications of Superposition

Quantum superposition is not just a philosophical puzzle; it has significant practical implications, especially in the emerging field of quantum computing. In a quantum computer, information bits, called qubits, can exist simultaneously in multiple states thanks to superposition. This allows quantum computers to process vast amounts of data and perform calculations at a speed and complexity that classical computers cannot match.

Together, uncertainty and superposition represent fundamental concepts that challenge our traditional conceptions of reality and causality. They provide the foundation on which not only advanced scientific theories are built but also revolutionary technologies that could define the future of computing, cryptography, and information theory. Understanding and applying these principles will continue to be at the forefront of scientific inquiry in the quest to unlock further secrets of the quantum universe.

Quantum Entanglement

Quantum entanglement is one of the most fascinating and mysterious phenomena of quantum physics. It describes a condition in which two or more particles become so deeply linked that the state of a single particle is instantaneously correlated with the state of the others, regardless of the distance separating them. This correlation not only challenges our traditional conceptions of space and time but also raises profound questions about the nature of reality itself.

Origins and Development of the Concept

The idea of quantum entanglement was first introduced by physicist Erwin Schrödinger in the 1930s as part of the debate over the interpretation of quantum mechanics. Albert Einstein, Boris Podolsky, and Nathan Rosen proposed the now-famous EPR (Einstein-Podolsky-Rosen) Paradox, through which they sought to demonstrate that quantum mechanics was incomplete. They believed that the phenomenon of entanglement implied the existence of as-yet-undiscovered "hidden variables" in quantum physics. Einstein described entanglement as "spooky action at a distance," expressing his discomfort with a concept that seemed to violate the principles of relativity, which assert that no information can travel faster than light.

Entanglement in Action

In practice, if two particles are entangled, measuring the state of one particle (such as position, velocity, polarization) will immediately determine the state of the other particle, no matter how distant it is. This occurs seemingly instantaneously, without any visible physical signal traveling between them. Experiments have repeatedly confirmed that entanglement works even when the entangled particles are separated by large distances, thus challenging the idea that information must travel through space to be communicated.

Philosophical and Scientific Implications

Quantum entanglement has significant philosophical implications, challenging our ideas about causality and locality. The ability of particles to instantaneously influence each other over large distances suggests that at the quantum level, the concept of "distance" may be very different from how we normally understand it. This has led some physicists to speculate about the possibility of an underlying substrate of reality where particles remain connected, a kind of quantum spacetime that eludes our current understanding.

Practical Applications

On a practical level, quantum entanglement is at the heart of emerging technologies in the field of quantum information, such as quantum computing and quantum cryptography. For example, quantum cryptography uses entanglement to create encryption keys that are practically impossible to decipher using traditional methods. In quantum computing, entanglement is used to vastly increase computing power compared to classical computers, allowing for calculations that would be virtually unfeasible otherwise.

Quantum entanglement remains one of the greatest mysteries and at the same time one of the greatest promises of modern physics. With its potential to revolutionize our information systems and our understanding of the universe, it continues to be a fertile field for scientific and philosophical exploration. The challenge of fully deciphering this phenomenon could ultimately lead to a new revolution in science, comparable to the revolution that quantum theory itself unleashed more than a century ago.

Implications of Quantum Reality

The implications of quantum reality are profound and varied, extending from the field of physics to philosophy, from technology to computer science. In the technological world, quantum theory underpins revolutionary innovations such as quantum computers, which promise to surpass the limits of classical computers using states of superposition and entanglement to perform calculations at previously unimaginable speeds.

Conclusion

Exploring the foundations of quantum reality represents a transformative journey not only for physics but for the entire realm of human knowledge. This field of study not only deepens our understanding of the universe at the subatomic level but also raises fundamental questions that touch on philosophy, metaphysics, and technology. Through this study, we are constantly compelled to reconsider and redefine our most deeply rooted conceptions about the nature of reality.

Reassessment of Fundamental Notions

Quantum reality forces us to question some of the most

elementary principles of the physical world. Concepts such as locality, causality, and even reality itself are revisited in light of the bizarre yet empirically verified properties of quantum particles. This has profound implications not only for how we understand the universe but also for how we interact with it on practical and theoretical levels.

Impact on Emerging Technologies

As we progress in the exploration of quantum mechanics, new doors constantly open for the development of revolutionary technologies. Quantum computing and quantum cryptography are just two examples of how the strange properties of quantum particles can be harnessed to make advances that were unimaginable with technologies based on classical physics. These technologies not only promise to accelerate computation and improve communication security but also to advance research in fields such as medicine and materials science by their ability to simulate complex molecular and chemical systems with unprecedented precision.

New Theories and Perspectives

The ongoing investigation into the field of quantum reality also stimulates the development of new theories that seek to unify quantum physics with general relativity and other areas of physics. These theories may one day provide a more complete and coherent description of the universe. Furthermore, the challenge of correctly interpreting quantum phenomena pushes philosophers and theorists to explore new modes of thinking about time, space, and the interconnectedness of all that exists.

Infinite Potential for Science and Philosophy

Finally, quantum reality remains a field of immeasurable value for science and philosophy. By continuing to explore and experiment, we keep the doors open to infinite possibilities of discovery and innovation. This ongoing expansion of our understanding not only empowers humanity's technological and scientific capabilities but also enriches our philosophical view of the world, inviting us to consider a reality much more intricate and interconnected than initially imagined. Studying quantum reality is therefore much more than an academic exploration; it is an adventure that rewrites the rules of reality and invites us to imagine new worlds, new existences, and new ways of being in an extraordinarily more complex and wonderfully mysterious universe.

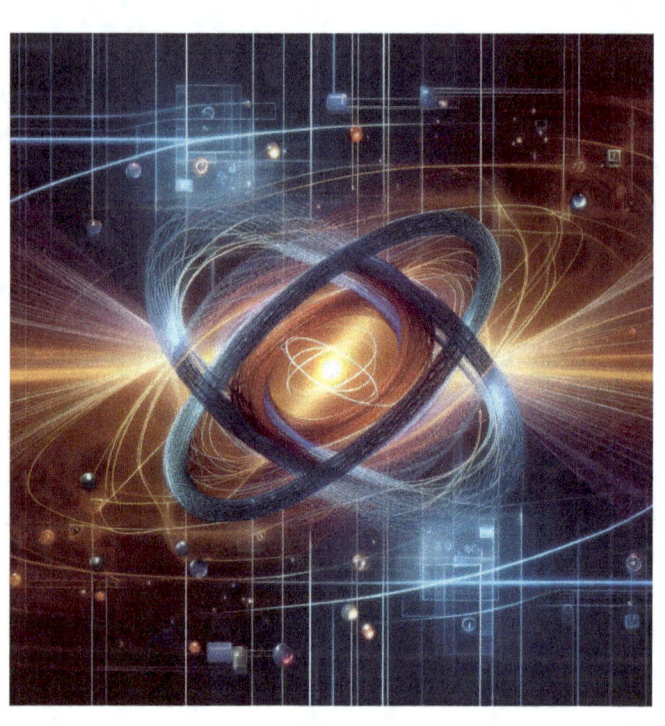

HOW QUANTUM PHYSICS APPLIES TO MANIFESTATION

Quantum physics, with its surprising and paradoxical discoveries, has opened new horizons not only in the field of science but also in personal and spiritual development. Particularly, the application of quantum mechanics principles to the concept of manifestation offers a fascinating and profoundly innovative view of how we can consciously influence the reality around us.

Fundamental Principles of Quantum Mechanics in Manifestation

Quantum mechanics revolutionizes our understanding of reality through a series of principles that challenge the laws of classical physics. At the core of these principles lies the concept of superposition, which introduces a view of reality as a canvas of potential rather than of defined and inevitable events.

Quantum Superposition and Reality as Potentiality

The principle of superposition is one of the fundamental pillars of quantum mechanics. It states that, at the subatomic level, particles like electrons do not exist in a single, definite state until measured. Instead, they exist in all possible states simultaneously, described by a wave function representing a probability distribution of all possible states the particle could be found in.

This principle is best illustrated in the famous double-slit experiment: when electrons are fired at a barrier with two slits, they do not pass through one slit or the other, but through both simultaneously, interfering with themselves as waves, creating an interference pattern on the detector that is characteristic of waves rather than particles. This phenomenon occurs only when there is no direct observation of the slits; mere observation collapses the wave function into a particular state.

Manifestation and the Observer's Influence

This approach to reality has profound implications for the concept of manifestation. If reality is a superposition of all possible states until observed, then the act of observation becomes an act of creation. Our intentions, expectations, and observations are not simply passive recordings of an external universe, but active participations that help define how that reality manifests.

In practice, this suggests that our intentions and attentions can influence the manifestation of reality in specific ways. When we focus our attention or intention on a particular state of affairs, we may be, in a sense, collapsing the universe's wave function around that possibility. This implies that maintaining a clear and consistent intention could physically influence the events and circumstances of our lives.

Ethical and Personal Implications of Quantum Manifestation

If we accept that our awareness and intentions can influence reality, significant ethical questions also arise. This power implies responsibility: the quality of our intentions and the purity of our attention become crucial. It's not just a matter of getting what we want but deeply aligning those desires with higher values and purposes.

Ultimately, integrating the principles of quantum mechanics into the practice of manifestation offers us a powerful and challenging perspective on how we might interact with and influence the world around us. This quantum view not only expands our concept of possibility but also invites us to deeply reflect on the nature of reality and our place and role within it. As co-creators in a dynamic and interactive universe, we have the opportunity—and perhaps even the obligation—to shape our reality with awareness, intention, and responsibility.

The Observer and Reality

The role of the observer in quantum mechanics introduces a radically new view of how perception and reality can be intertwined. This concept, often illustrated through the double-slit experiment, not only underscores the intrinsic ambiguity of the subatomic nature but also opens doors to a deeper understanding of the power of human observation.

The Double-Slit Experiment and the Observer Effect

In the double-slit experiment, particles like photons or electrons are fired at a barrier with two apertures. If there is no observation of which slit the particles pass through, they exhibit wave-like behavior, interfering with themselves and forming an interference pattern on the detection screen behind the slits. However, if one decides to measure which slit the particles pass through, they suddenly cease to behave like waves, and their paths become those of discrete particles, eliminating the interference pattern.

This phenomenon shows that the behavior of matter at the quantum level can be altered by the mere presence of an observer, or more precisely, by the act of measurement. This behavior has led to the formulation of one of the most intriguing principles of quantum physics: reality at this level exists in a state of superposition until the moment of observation, which "collapses" this superposition into a particular state.

Philosophical Implications of the Observer Effect

The observer effect challenges our traditional notions of objectivity and reality. If the act of observation can alter the outcome of an experiment, then to what extent is reality independent of the observer? This question has profound philosophical implications, leading some to speculate that reality may not be a fixed and immutable structure, but rather a dynamic fabric influenced by our perceptions, intentions, and consciousness.

Manifestation and Co-Creation of Reality

Applying these principles to manifestation reveals a powerful vision of reality as something we can actively co-shape. If our observations can influence the behavior of particles at the quantum level, it is plausible to think that intentional and conscious focus can influence our physical and experiential reality. Our expectations, beliefs, and intentions, therefore, are not merely passive reactions to events but actively participate in shaping the environment around us.

This understanding radically transforms how we perceive our role in the universe. We are no longer simple passive observers but active participants in shaping our world. Awareness of this power carries great responsibility: it invites us to carefully consider what intentions we bring into our daily lives and how these intentions might shape not only our lives but also the world around us.

Ultimately, the role of the observer in quantum physics not only deepens our understanding of matter and energy but also offers a revolutionary paradigm for understanding our personal and collective power of manifestation. Embracing this role, we can begin to see ourselves as active co-creators, consciously using our focus to positively influence and shape the reality we experience every day.

Quantum Entanglement and Universal Connection

Quantum entanglement, which describes how separated particles can instantaneously influence each other over even vast distances, provides another powerful metaphor for manifestation. This "entanglement" suggests that all parts of the universe are connected in a subtle and interdependent web, where actions or events in one place can have immediate repercussions elsewhere.

For those practicing manifestation, entanglement can be seen as a reminder of the profound interconnection between ourselves and the universe around us. Our intentions and thoughts are not isolated but are part of a dynamic network of interactions that can be shaped to facilitate desired outcomes. This reinforces the idea of a responsive and participatory universe, where reality can be influenced through careful and conscious positioning of thoughts and intentions.

Conscious Manifestation and the Challenge of Quantum Coherence

In the field of manifestation, the concept of quantum coherence, where quantum systems can exist in states of interference that make them incredibly sensitive to external disturbances, can be likened to the need to maintain coherence and alignment in our intentions. Coherence in our thoughts and feelings can enhance our ability to positively influence our reality, much like how a cohesive quantum system can perform complex and powerful operations.

Conclusion

Applying the principles of quantum physics to the practice of manifestation offers a powerful paradigm through which we can understand our role in shaping our reality. It invites us to more deeply consider the power of our intentions, the importance of our attention, and the profound implication that we are, at every moment, actively involved in creating the fabric of our experience. This perspective not only enriches our understanding of manifestation but also broadens our sense of responsibility and possibility in the vast, interconnected theater of existence.

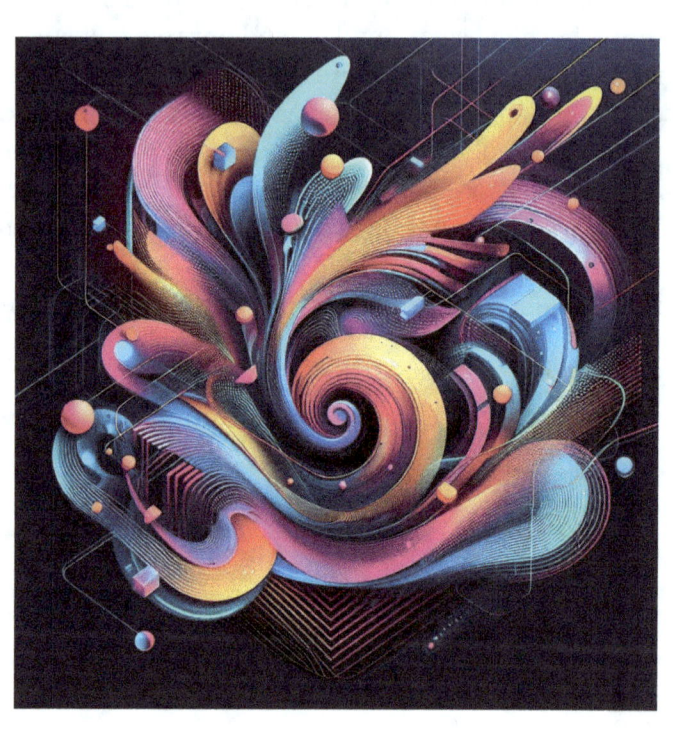

THE MIND-UNIVERSE CONNECTION

The Role of Consciousness in Shaping Reality

The connection between mind and universe is one of the most fascinating and complex themes at the intersection of quantum physics, philosophy, and metaphysics. This relationship underscores a fundamental question: to what extent does human consciousness influence external reality? Delving into this question leads to reflections on how our perceptions, thoughts, and intentions can not only interpret but actually shape the very fabric of reality.

Consciousness as an Agent of Reality

Quantum physics, with its revolutionary discoveries, has radically altered conventional understanding of the universe. One of the most intriguing aspects of this science is the proactive role that consciousness appears to play in shaping reality itself. Through phenomena like the observer effect and quantum superposition, new perspectives emerge on how observation and measurement are not mere passive acts, but interactions that can actually determine the structure and behavior of reality at the microscopic level.

Implications of the Active Role of Consciousness

According to quantum mechanics, particles such as electrons and photons exist in a state of superposition, manifesting a range of potential locations, velocities, and other properties until the moment of observation. It is the act of observation itself, according to the principle of superposition, that "collapses" these different potentials into a single observable state. This process not only underscores the fluidity of physical reality but also implies that the observer's consciousness actively participates in determining how and in what state these potentials manifest.

The idea that consciousness can influence reality extends beyond mere observation. The context, expectations, beliefs, and even the intentions of the observer can alter the outcome of quantum experiments. This concept has been demonstrated in various experiments, where different observers obtain different results, not only due to random variability but also due to differences in their expectations and methodological approach.

Implications for Understanding the Universe

These discoveries raise fundamental questions about the nature of reality and the relationship between mind and matter. If consciousness can influence reality at the quantum level, this might suggest that the fundamental properties of the universe are accessible and modifiable through mental processes. This leads to speculation that reality itself may be less an objective given and more an emergent construct from interactions between individual consciousness and the laws of physics.

Continued Research and Exploration

This conception of consciousness as an agent of reality has spurred a vast field of interdisciplinary research. Scientists are investigating how these principles can be applied in practical contexts, exploring potential impacts in technology, medicine, and psychology. Additionally, the convergence of quantum physics and spiritual and meditative approaches to reality suggests innovative and more integrated ways of exploring the relationship between mind and universe.

In summary, the perspective of consciousness as an agent of reality not only challenges our way of thinking about physics but also offers a richer and more dynamic view of our role in the universe. With each new experiment and theory, we move closer to a deeper understanding of how our perception and participation can shape not only our understanding of reality but reality itself.

Philosophical Implications of the Mind-Universe Connection

The perspective that the mind can actively influence reality introduces a conceptual revolution that profoundly challenges traditional paradigms of causality and the perception of an external universe independent of our consciousness. This notion, drawing from the principles of quantum physics, raises fundamental questions about the nature of reality and the relationship between consciousness and the physical world.

Reconsideration of Causality

Classical causality, based on a linear relationship of cause and effect, is called into question by the possibility that consciousness can influence or determine the state of physical reality. If the act of observation can change the outcome of a quantum event, then the unidirectional flow from cause to effect is complicated by a feedback loop in which consciousness is not just a passive receiver but an active participant in reality creation. This raises questions about the nature of time, sequentiality, and simultaneity of events.

Independence of the External World

The conception of an objective external world independent of human perception is another fundamental concept that is challenged. If consciousness can alter the state of matter at the quantum level, then the distinction between observing subject and observed object becomes less defined. This suggests a more holistic and interconnected reality, where the separation between mind and matter, internal and external, fades into a dynamic continuum of interaction and co-creation.

Realism versus Idealism

The potential influence of the mind on reality reignites the philosophical debate between realism and idealism. While realism posits the existence of an external world independent of human perception, idealism proposes that reality is somehow constituted or mediated by consciousness. If reality is partly co-created by our perception and cognition, we move closer to an idealistic view of the universe, where consciousness is not an epiphenomenon but a fundamental element of the structure of reality.

Matter, Space, and Time as Mental Constructs

The possibility that matter, space, and time are influenced or even derived from consciousness raises questions about the fundamental nature of existence. If these basic elements of reality can be modulated or conditioned by perception, then our understanding of the universe and our own existence requires a deeper exploration of the dynamics between mind and matter. This perspective paves the way for a more integrated and unitary approach to science, philosophy, and spirituality, suggesting that the pursuit of truth requires a synthesis of external investigations and inner introspections.

The philosophical implications of the mind-universe connection challenge our existing models of reality, inviting us to explore new dimensions of human understanding. This inquiry not only enriches our knowledge but also invites us to reconsider our role in the fabric of existence, offering us a more participatory and co-creative view of the universe in which we live.

Dynamic Interactions between Mind and Matter

The idea of a participatory universe, where observers and the observed system are intertwined in continuous dialogue, offers a new way of conceiving science and spirituality. In this view, the human mind assumes an active role in shaping reality through processes that include meditation, mindful intention, and visualization. These practices, once confined to the fringes of science, are now being studied for their potential to influence physical health, mental performance, and even material outcomes.

Human Potential in a Responsive Universe

The possibility that the human mind can interact with the universe in meaningful and profound ways not only transforms our understanding of our place in the cosmos but also opens up revolutionary scenarios for exploring human potential. This interaction is not limited to simple passive perception or reaction to external events but extends to active and deliberate participation in reality shaping.

Beyond Perception and Reaction

Traditionally, humans are thought to perceive the world through the senses and react based on this perception. However, if consciousness can actively influence reality, as some principles of quantum physics suggest, then the possibility of a much more active role opens up: that of co-creators of reality. In this context, humans are not just responding to stimuli but using their awareness, intentions, and cognitive abilities to actively influence and shape their environment.

Active Participation in Reality Creation

The conception of a responsive universe, where every thought and intention can leave a tangible imprint, underscores the importance of conscious participation in the dynamics of life. This means that every decision made, every goal pursued, and every dream nurtured can have direct and measurable effects not only on individuals but on the entire fabric of social and environmental reality.

Responsibility and Creative Potential

With this great ability to influence comes a correspondingly great responsibility. If every thought and intention has the potential to shape reality, then it becomes imperative that we engage in positive reflections and actions aimed at creating a desirable future for all. This responsibility urges individuals to carefully consider the long-term consequences of their actions and cultivate a mindset oriented not only toward personal success but also toward collective well-being.

Development of Human and Technological Capacities

The acceptance of the idea that we can co-create our reality also stimulates the development of new capacities and technologies. For example, meditation and visualization techniques could be further developed and integrated with advanced technological tools to enhance the effectiveness with which we influence reality. This directly connects to the development of augmented and virtual reality technologies, which can be used as extensions of our ability to model environments and scenarios, not only digitally but also in the physical world.

Realizing human potential in a responsive universe requires a new way of thinking about who we are and how we interact with the world around us. We are no longer just passive spectators; we are active participants with the ability to influence and shape our environment in ways we could only imagine before. This new paradigm not only enriches our sense of agency and purpose but also invites us to live with an awareness and intentionality that reflect our power to co-create reality.

Conclusion

The mind-universe connection, therefore, is not just a topic of theoretical speculation but a gateway to new dimensions of reality and human existence. Exploring and understanding this connection not only enriches our understanding of reality but also expands our ability to consciously interact with the world, suggesting that our consciousness and creativity are powerful forces that can literally shape the universe in which we live.

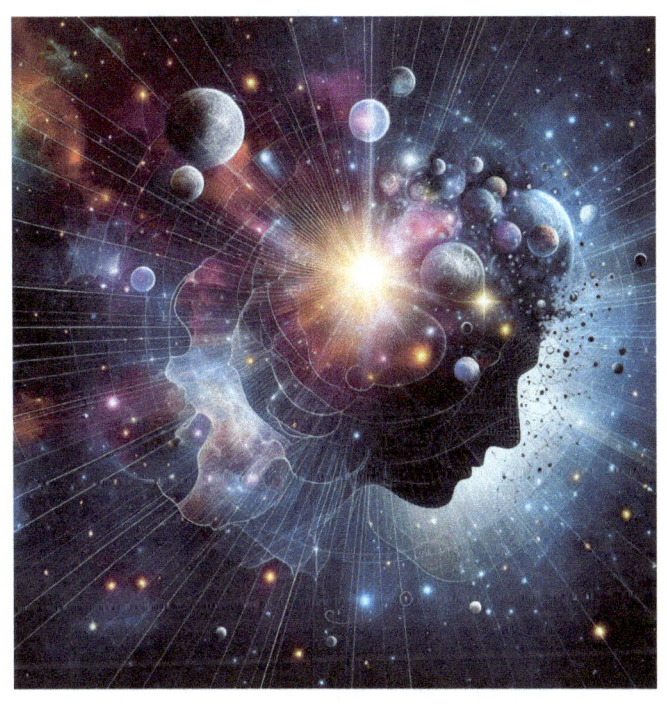

PRINCIPLES OF SYNCHRONICITY AND CONNECTION

EXAMPLES OF HOW INTENTION INFLUENCES THE ENVIRONMENT

The concept of synchronicity, introduced by Carl Jung, refers to the simultaneous occurrence of two events that are not causally connected but whose relationship is meaningful to those who perceive them. This principle, combined with the idea of the intrinsic connection between intention and the environment, offers us a profound framework for exploring how our intentions can influence the reality that surrounds us.

Definition of Synchronicity and Connection

The concept of synchronicity, initially introduced by Carl Jung, refers to the peculiarity of external events that, although not causally linked, manifest in ways that deeply resonate with an individual's internal state. These events, which may seem merely coincidental, are often experienced with an intensity that suggests a deeper and more significant connection.

Synchronicity as Alignment between Internal and External

Synchronicity occurs when there is alignment between an

individual's internal dynamics—their thoughts, emotions, expectations, or desires—and events in the external world. This alignment is perceived as highly significant by the subject experiencing it, transforming an apparent coincidence into an event laden with personal meaning. Such experiences challenge the idea of a reality governed solely by cause-and-effect relationships and suggest the possibility of a more complex fabric of reality, where scientifically immeasurable factors have a direct impact on event manifestation.

Synchronicity and the Network of Subtle Relationships

Synchronicity not only implies the manifestation of significant coincidences but also emphasizes the presence of a network of subtle relationships that interconnect the individual with the surrounding environment in ways that transcend ordinary understanding of physics. This suggests that the universe operates not only on principles of linear causality but also includes dimensions of interaction that reflect a sort of implicit order or holistic connectivity. In this context, intentions, desires, and thoughts can influence external reality, intertwining with events in ways that favor the occurrence of synchronicity.

Implications of Synchronicity in Daily Life

These moments of deep connection can have a transformative impact on an individual's life. The perception that the universe can somehow respond to our internal states can profoundly influence our way of perceiving ourselves and the world, offering a view of reality in which we are active participants rather than passive observers. This perception can lead to a renewed sense of purpose and agency, encouraging individuals to cultivate thoughts and intentions that reflect their deepest goals and desires, with the hope that such internal orientations may manifest in synchronistic external events.

In conclusion, synchronicity as a concept and experience underlines a worldview in which the barriers between internal and external are less defined, and where our lives are woven into a fabric of reality that responds in mysterious but often meaningful ways. This concept not only enriches our experience of life with a dimension of magic and mystery but also raises stimulating questions about the true capabilities of the human mind and the nature of our universe.

Influence of Intention on the Environment

Intention is a powerful force that appears to play a crucial role in shaping our environment. Various theories and practices suggest that when people focus their attention consistently and purposefully, they can experience results that seem to defy statistical probability. Here are some examples:

1. **Effects of Group Meditation**:

Studies have explored how group meditation can influence social and environmental variables. Events like "the Global Coherence Project" have shown that large groups of people meditating together with the intention of reducing conflict or increasing peace can correlate with a reduction in violence and an increase in cooperation in specific geographical areas.

2. **Experiments on Living Systems**:

Research has demonstrated that intentions can influence plant growth, the formation of water crystals, and even animal behavior. For example, in experiments where individuals projected positive intentions toward water samples, changes in the molecular structure of the water were observed, as documented in the famous experiments by Dr. Masaru Emoto.

3. **Manifestation and Personal Synchronicity**:

Many people report experiences where specific intentions seem to attract circumstances, encounters, or information that are perfectly aligned with their desires or needs, even in unexpected ways. These episodes of synchronicity not only confirm their intentions but often provide the resources or encounters necessary to realize their goals.

Field Theories and Connectivity

Some contemporary theories in physics suggest that these manifestations of synchronicity can be explained through concepts such as morphogenetic fields or networks of quantum information, which describe how intention can interact with a field of energy and information that connects all entities in the universe. These theories propose that human intention can modulate and influence this field, leading to concrete manifestations in the physical world.

Conclusion

The principles of synchronicity and connection invite us to reflect on the interdependence between ourselves and the universe that surrounds us. They challenge our understanding of reality and broaden our perception of human possibilities, suggesting that through consciousness and intention, we are capable of co-creating and significantly influencing the fabric of our existence. This recognition opens not only new avenues of scientific research but also personal practices that can enrich our daily lives and our impact on the world.

LESSONS FROM DOLORES CANNON

CANNON'S MAIN DISCOVERIES AND THEORIES

Dolores Cannon, a pioneer in the field of regression hypnosis and past-life research, has left an indelible mark through her unique work and revolutionary theories. Her hypnosis techniques, collectively known as the Quantum Healing Hypnosis Technique (QHHT), and her discoveries in the fields of spiritual healing, past lives, and esoteric cosmology have opened new doors to understanding human existence and the universe.

Quantum Healing Hypnosis Technique (QHHT)

The Quantum Healing Hypnosis Technique (QHHT) is a pioneering method of regression hypnosis developed by Dolores Cannon, which revolutionized the field of hypnotic therapies. The technique is based on the premise that accessing a state of superconsciousness, or the "superconscious mind," allows individuals to explore not only past-life memories but also to connect with the deep and universal wisdom that resides within every human being.

Induction into a State of Deep Trance

At the heart of QHHT is the induction of the subject into a state of deep trance. This state, different from ordinary levels of consciousness or sleep, allows individuals to transcend the barriers of the conscious mind and access those parts of the subconscious normally inaccessible in everyday life. Dolores Cannon believed that in this state, subjects are capable of transcending the boundaries of time and space to access experiences and memories that transcend their current physical existence.

Exploration of Past Lives

QHHT distinguishes itself for its structured approach to exploring past lives. Cannon used this technique to guide subjects through a detailed journey into their previous existences, retrieving memories often buried deep in the subconscious. These sessions are not just narratives of past events but are also experiences rich in emotions and sensations that, according to Cannon, carry the keys to understanding and resolving current physical and emotional issues.

Physical and Emotional Healing

One of the most innovative aspects of QHHT is its use of retrieved information to facilitate deep healing. According to Cannon, many physical illnesses and emotional distress have roots in traumas or unresolved issues from past lives. Through QHHT, subjects can identify these ingrained causes and work on them, not only on a psychological level but also on an energetic level, often resulting in significant improvements or complete healing.

Insights into Health, Relationships, and Spiritual Obstacles

QHHT sessions often offer valuable insights into a wide range of personal issues, including current health problems, relational dynamics, and spiritual obstacles. These revelations provide subjects with a deeper understanding of their challenges and the karmic dynamics or lessons that may lie at their core. With this knowledge, subjects are often able to make more informed and conscious choices in their daily lives, thereby improving their quality of life and overall well-being.

In summary, Dolores Cannon's Quantum Healing Hypnosis Technique is not just a methodology for exploring past lives but a powerful tool for personal transformation. Through QHHT, individuals have the opportunity to connect with the deepest and wisest part of themselves, bringing to light and resolving ancient issues and catalyzing a process of healing and understanding that goes far beyond the conventional.

Theories on Past Lives

Dolores Cannon, through her pioneering work with the Quantum Healing Hypnosis Technique (QHHT), has significantly contributed to the understanding of past lives, a central theme in esoteric sciences. Her extensive research has opened new horizons in the understanding of reincarnation and the spiritual evolution of souls.

Detailed Exploration of Past Lives

The QHHT sessions conducted by Cannon have allowed for detailed narratives of past existences, not only terrestrial but also extraterrestrial. These narratives often included descriptions of civilizations on other planets and in other dimensions, offering an expanded and radical view of soul existence beyond earthly boundaries. These accounts not only enrich our understanding of the universe but also broaden the perspective on existential possibilities beyond life on Earth.

The Reincarnation and Evolution of Souls

According to Cannon, souls do not reincarnate in isolation; rather, they go through a series of bodily lives to experience a wide range of circumstances, which help them evolve and mature spiritually. This evolution is seen not only as an individual process but as a shared journey with groups of souls, often referred to as "soul families." These groups reincarnate together repeatedly, assuming various roles in different lives to help each other learn and grow through different experiences and challenges.

Influence of Past Lives on Present Life

Cannon explored how the dynamics and lessons of past lives can have a direct impact on the interactions and challenges of present life. For example, an unresolved conflict in a past life might manifest as relational tension in the present life, or an unexplainable fear might have roots in traumas from past lives. Understanding these connections offers subjects the opportunity to resolve these issues through healing and introspection, often resulting in emotional releases and significant personal transformations.

Karmic Lessons and Spiritual Growth

Cannon's approach also emphasizes the concept of karmic lessons: the challenges and situations that a soul encounters in a life are often shaped to teach specific spiritual lessons necessary for its evolution. This view suggests that events in our lives are not random but are intrinsically designed to guide us towards greater awareness and spiritual understanding. Accessing memories of past lives can thus serve as a valuable tool for deciphering the deeper meaning behind the experiences of our current life.

In summary, Dolores Cannon's theories on past lives not only enrich the field of esoteric sciences with detailed and complex narratives but also offer a transformative perspective on the nature of life and spiritual development. These teachings continue to influence and inspire many who seek a deeper understanding of their existence and spiritual path, highlighting how the discovery of our past can illuminate our present and guide us towards a more conscious and fulfilled future.

Interactions with Non-Terrestrial Entities

Among Cannon's most controversial findings are her claims regarding human interactions with non-terrestrial entities. Through QHHT sessions, many of her clients have reported encounters with extraterrestrial beings and described complex cosmic narratives involving alien civilizations and their impact on human history. Cannon theorized that these interactions are part of a vast cosmic plan of evolution and assistance, in which extraterrestrial beings act as guides or teachers to help humanity in its spiritual growth.

Implications of Cannon's Discoveries

Dolores Cannon's discoveries, through her pioneering work with the Quantum Healing Hypnosis Technique (QHHT), have led to a radical reconsideration of many of our traditional conceptions about the universe and reality. Her research has revealed a complexity and interconnectedness of existence that far exceeds the materialistic and mechanistic interpretations traditionally accepted.

Challenging Conventional Conceptions of Reality

Cannon discovered that reality, far from being a mere static backdrop for human activity, is a dynamic field of possibilities that constantly interacts with human consciousness. Her QHHT sessions have shown that individuals can access information that is not limited by time or space. These findings suggest that our standard understanding of time as sequential and space as fixed may be only a useful convention rather than an absolute truth about the nature of the world.

Complexity and Interconnection of the Universe

The narratives of past lives and experiences reported by Cannon's clients illustrate a universe in which multiple lives and parallel dimensions are interconnected in ways that defy linear logic. This view of reality as an intricate network of mutual influences between past, present, and future, as well as between different dimensional realities, significantly broadens the scope of our existence.

Transcending the Limits of Time and Space

One of the most revolutionary aspects of Cannon's discoveries is the idea that human consciousness can transcend the boundaries of time and space. Testimonies from subjects in deep trance states indicate that people can live and perceive events beyond their immediate spatiotemporal context, suggesting that the mind and consciousness are not bound by the physical restrictions we have assumed were universal.

Exploration of Realms beyond Materialistic Understanding

Cannon's discoveries open the door to explorations of

realms that conventional science has often relegated to the margins or completely ignored. The implications of such discoveries are vast, leading to the consideration of non-material realities as an integral part of our existence. This invites a broader examination of human potentialities and the true nature of the universe, prompting scientists, philosophers, and spiritual researchers to consider new dimensions of human exploration.

Ultimately, Dolores Cannon's discoveries not only challenge our conventional perceptions but also invite a deeper and more integrated understanding of reality. What emerges is a framework of existence that is infinitely richer and more complex than most have ever considered. These ideas have the potential to transform not only how we see ourselves and our place in the universe but also how we approach the big questions about life, consciousness, and the continuity of existence itself.

Conclusion

Dolores Cannon's teachings continue to influence and inspire those who seek a deeper understanding of human existence and its connections with the wider universe. Her theories and methods open new paths for personal understanding and healing, inviting each individual to explore the depths of their own soul and consider the limitless possibilities that existence has to offer.

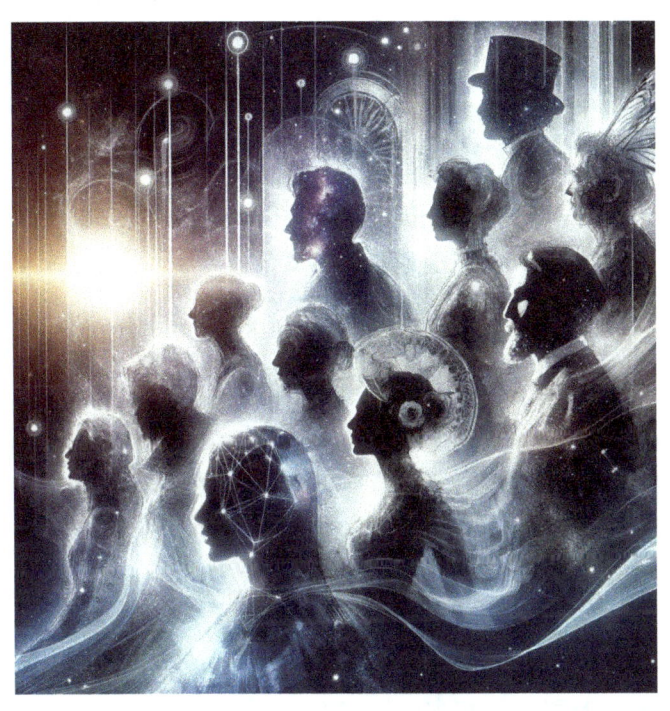

SUMMARY OF DOLORES CANNON'S MOST INFLUENTIAL DISCOVERIES

Dolores Cannon, through decades of research and clinical practice in the field of regression hypnosis, has contributed a series of discoveries that have profoundly influenced the field of esoteric sciences and spiritual healing. Her techniques and the results obtained have not only expanded the understanding of human soul dynamics but have also opened new pathways for understanding time, space, and non-physical dimensions.

Quantum Healing Hypnosis Technique (QHHT)

The creation of QHHT represents one of her most notable contributions. This technique allows subjects to access what Cannon termed the state of "superconscious mind," where profound revelations and transformations are possible. Using QHHT, Cannon has guided thousands of people through a process that not only allows exploration of past lives but also facilitates physical and psychological healings often described as miraculous by participants.

Discoveries on Past Lives

The detailed narratives of past lives collected by Cannon have provided an unprecedented view of the cyclical nature of human existence. The stories gathered range from earthly existences to incarnations in other worlds and dimensions, suggesting a universe where souls travel through different states of being to learn, evolve, and grow. These discoveries have significantly expanded our understanding of reincarnation and spiritual evolution.

Theories on Soul Groups

Another revolutionary concept introduced by Cannon is that of soul groups, or soul families, reincarnating together. This has offered a new lens through which to view personal relationships and family ties, suggesting that our connections with others may have roots that extend far beyond a single lifetime. This idea has provided comfort and understanding to many, offering a broader perspective on relational dynamics and personal difficulties.

Interactions with Non-Terrestrial Entities

Perhaps among the most daring have been her claims and discoveries regarding interactions between humans and non-terrestrial entities. Through QHHT sessions, Cannon documented numerous cases of individuals reporting detailed interactions with alien civilizations. These narratives not only challenge our understanding of the universe but also broaden the context in which we can consider our existence and technological and spiritual development.

Impact on Contemporary Thought

Cannon's theories and discoveries have inspired a wave of reflection among psychologists, healers, scientists, and spiritual researchers, influencing a wide range of disciplines. The implications of her discoveries continue to stimulate debate on fundamental issues such as the nature of consciousness, the role of the soul in healing, and the structure of time and space.

Conclusion

In summary, Dolores Cannon's work remains a milestone in the field of consciousness research and human existence beyond material boundaries. Her discoveries not only challenge but enrich our knowledge landscape, offering new ways of thinking about life, healing, and universal interconnectedness. Her legacy continues to influence and inspire, promising to fuel further explorations and discoveries in the fields of science and spirituality.

APPLICATION OF D. CANNON'S TECHNIQUES IN EVERYDAY LIFE

The regression and healing techniques developed by Dolores Cannon, particularly the Quantum Healing Hypnosis Technique (QHHT), not only provide insights into understanding the dynamics of past lives but also offer practical tools that can be integrated into everyday life. This practical guide explores how Cannon's methods can be applied to enhance personal well-being and promote ongoing spiritual growth.

Integration of Past Awareness into Present Life

1. **Personal Reflection and Meditation**:

Before applying regression techniques, it is helpful to develop a regular meditation practice. This helps calm the mind and prepares the individual to receive deeper insights during self-exploration or guided regression sessions. Daily meditation can help maintain a connection with one's higher self, which according to Cannon, is a source of wisdom and guidance.

2. **Synchronicity Journal**:

Dolores Cannon emphasized the importance of synchronicities as messages from the universe. Keeping a journal of synchronicities and significant coincidences can help recognize and interpret signals that may be connected to lessons from past lives or insights into the current life path.

Use of Regressions for Healing and Introspection

1. Self-Hypnosis Sessions:

While QHHT is generally conducted by a certified therapist, individuals can explore self-hypnosis techniques that incorporate some basic principles of QHHT to explore their own past lives. This may include guided visualizations that encourage the individual to imagine themselves in other times and places, seeking insights or resolutions to current issues.

2. Application of Past Lessons:

Utilize the information obtained from regression sessions to address present issues. For example, if a regression reveals that a fear or problem has roots in a past life, consciously working to resolve these issues in the present can lead to significant emotional and spiritual healing.

Development of an Empathic Connection with Others

1. Recognition of Ancestral and Karmic Connections:

Cannon's discoveries about soul families may encourage individuals to consider present relationships in a new light. Understanding that certain bonds may have deep roots can help develop greater empathy and patience in interpersonal relationships.

2. **Sharing and Support in the Healing Journey**:

Forming support groups or participating in workshops on regression techniques can provide a platform for sharing and mutual learning. These groups can offer a space to share experiences and insights gained through the application of Cannon's methods, thus facilitating a journey of collective healing.

Conclusion

Dolores Cannon's techniques, when applied in everyday life, not only offer the opportunity to explore the depths of our souls but also to live a more conscious and fulfilling life. Integrating these methods can help individuals connect with a broader wisdom, resolve internal conflicts, and navigate their lives with greater intentionality and spiritual understanding.

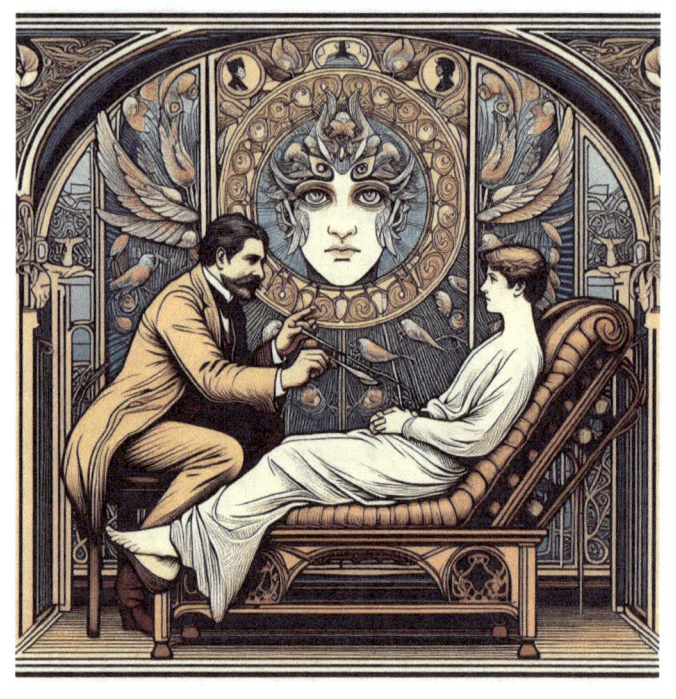

PREPARATION FOR MANIFESTATION

CLEANSING AND CLARIFICATION OF INTENTION

Inner Cleansing

1. **Identification and Release of Emotional Blocks**:
Identifying and releasing emotional blocks is a fundamental step in preparing for the manifestation of one's intentions. Before being able to start building new desired realities, it is essential to address and resolve old patterns and limiting beliefs that may hinder progress. These blocks can be unresolved fears, past disappointments or failures, or entrenched beliefs that are no longer in line with your current goals and desires.

The techniques for releasing these blocks are varied and can be adapted to individual needs. Meditation, for example, offers a space of tranquility and reflection where you can observe your thought patterns and emotions without judgment, allowing you to recognize those beliefs that serve more as obstacles than support to your well-being and development. Through regular meditation, you can gradually relax the grip of these limiting patterns and open the way to new possibilities.

Reflective writing is another powerful tool for emotional processing. Writing down your thoughts and emotions can help clarify inner issues and uncover roots of beliefs that may be buried under years of unconscious habits. This writing process can work as a dialogue with yourself, revealing authentic desires and areas of necessary transformation.

Additionally, working with a therapist can expedite this release process. A professional can offer expert guidance to navigate complex emotional labyrinths and provide support and specific strategies to address and resolve these blocks. Whether it's traditional therapy, spiritual counseling, or life coaching sessions, professional assistance can be incredibly effective in facilitating significant change.

Releasing emotional blocks is not a process that completes in a single moment; it may take time and constant practice. However, every step taken to overcome these obstacles not only frees up energy for new creations and manifestations but also contributes to a deeper understanding of oneself and a more fulfilling life authentically aligned with one's deepest desires.

2. **Environmental Purification**:

The physical environment can significantly influence the manifestation process. Creating a space that reflects aspirations and is free from clutter or objects that evoke negative energies or painful memories can facilitate a clearer and more powerful energy flow. Consider practicing decluttering, using feng shui, or purifying the space with sage or incense.

Clarification of Intentions

1. **Defining Clear and Measurable Goals**:

Intentions for manifestation play a crucial role in personal and professional realization processes. To be effective, these intentions must be formulated according to SMART criteria, meaning they must be Specific, Measurable, Achievable, Relevant, and Time-bound. This approach ensures that goals are not just vague wishes but well-defined action plans that can be effectively pursued and achieved.

Firstly, specific intentions eliminate ambiguity and allow for focusing energy on what truly matters. For example, rather than generically wishing for "success," it is more productive to specify what that success means in concrete terms, such as "achieving a promotion at work within six months" or "increasing the company's revenue by 20% by the end of the year."

Intentions should also be measurable, meaning there is a clear criterion for evaluating progress towards their achievement. This can include quantitative indicators like numbers or percentages, or qualitative indicators like achieving a certain skill level or completing a project.

Additionally, intentions should be achievable. Setting realistic goals that consider available resources, time, and personal circumstances is essential to maintaining motivation and avoiding frustration. An goal that seems out of reach can be discouraging, while one that is challenging but realistic can motivate and inspire.

Relevant intentions are those that resonate with your deepest values and align with your long-term aspirations. This alignment ensures that the time and energy invested in achieving the goals are a meaningful investment in your life, not just an item to check off a to-do list.

Finally, intentions must be time-bound, with clear and defined deadlines. Having a deadline helps structure the process and maintain the necessary urgency to take concrete actions. Without a deadline, goals may be continually postponed, reducing the likelihood of ever achieving them.

For example, instead of stating a generic desire for happiness, a more defined and SMART goal could be "I want to start a business that reflects my values by the end of the year." This not only specifies what you want to achieve but also includes a measure of success, alignment with personal values, the feasibility of starting a business within a defined timeframe, and a clear deadline that imposes a timeline for action.

2. **Creative Visualization**:

Once intentions are clarified, visualization can serve as a powerful tool to solidify these aspirations in consciousness. Dedicate time each day to vividly visualize oneself achieving the goals can reinforce the connection between desire and action. Imagining living the desired reality with all senses can amplify the effectiveness of manifestation.

3. **Positive Affirmations**:

Affirmations are positive statements that reinforce and activate intentions in daily life. Repeating these affirmations daily can help maintain focus on goals and promote a positive mental attitude open to opportunities.

Conclusion

Preparing for manifestation is a complex and dynamic process that goes far beyond simply formulating a wish. It requires active and deliberate commitment not only to identify and overcome obstacles that may hinder goal achievement but also to define personal aspirations and intentions precisely and clearly. This journey, which involves both clearing internal barriers such as fears and limiting beliefs and removing external obstacles, is crucial for creating the ideal conditions for realizing one's dreams.

Deepening Cleansing and Clarification

The cleansing process involves deep introspection and reflection. Recognizing and releasing old thought patterns or behaviors that no longer serve one's well-being can free up a significant amount of mental and emotional energy. This release not only helps to see one's true desires more clearly but also to take more effective actions towards them. Intention clarification, on the other hand, ensures that every step taken is aligned with the deepest values and authentic ambitions. Establishing clear and measurable goals with SMART criteria, as discussed earlier, is a crucial aspect of this process.

Impact on Personal and Spiritual Growth

In addition to facilitating the achievement of specific goals, adequate preparation for manifestation also has a profound impact on personal and spiritual growth.

Through this process, individuals often discover aspects of themselves that were previously hidden or suppressed. Facing and overcoming personal challenges can lead to greater self-awareness and self-understanding, elements that are essential for living a fulfilled and realized life.

Transformation of the Journey

When preparation for manifestation is approached with seriousness and dedication, the journey towards goal achievement becomes a transformative journey in itself. Every small success and every obstacle overcome builds confidence and resilience, qualities that are indispensable not only for manifestation but for all aspects of life. Furthermore, this process can strengthen the connection with one's higher self and with the universe, a relationship that many find enriching and comforting.

Ultimately, preparing for manifestation is not just a means to an end, but an opportunity to embark on a journey of personal discovery that can significantly enhance the quality of life. With the right commitment and appropriate techniques, it is possible not only to realize one's dreams but also to grow and evolve in ways that were unimaginable at the beginning of the journey.

TECHNIQUES FOR CLARIFYING AND PURIFYING INTENTIONS

Techniques for Clarifying and Purifying Intentions

Clarity and purity of intentions are essential for effective and meaningful manifestation. The process of clarifying and purifying intentions not only helps to focus desires and goals but also facilitates a deeper connection with the inner self and the universe. Let's explore some effective techniques that can be employed to refine and purify intentions.

1. Meditation and Inner Reflection

Meditation is a powerful tool for intention clarification. Practicing daily meditation helps to calm the mind and detach from the noise and distractions of everyday life, creating space for deeper internal reflection. Through meditation, one can access a state of expanded awareness where it becomes easier to identify and release limiting thoughts and beliefs. A specific technique is intention-focused meditation, where one meditates directly on the goal or desire, visualizing it clearly and nurturing positive energy around it.

2. Reflective Writing

Writing is another effective method for exploring and defining intentions. Keeping a journal where thoughts, feelings, and reflections are noted can reveal hidden thought patterns and help clarify what is truly desired. A useful technique is to write letters to oneself from the future, describing in detail the achievement of goals and the steps needed to get there. This exercise not only clarifies intentions but also increases motivation and commitment towards their attainment.

3. Positive Affirmations

Affirmations are positive statements repeated regularly to strengthen belief in one's abilities and the success of one's intentions. Creating and reciting specific affirmations daily that clearly reflect desired goals helps internalize these intentions and maintain a constant focus on them. It is important to formulate affirmations in positive terms and in the present tense, as if the goal has already been achieved, to enhance their effect on the subconscious.

4. Creative Visualization

Visualization is a powerful practice for cementing intentions in the subconscious mind. It involves mentally creating vivid images of oneself achieving desired goals. This process not only further clarifies intentions but also establishes an emotional connection with the goals, making manifestation more tangible and realistic.

5. Energetic Cleansing

Energetic cleansing can be achieved through various practices such as the use of sage, aromatherapy, salt baths, or Reiki sessions. These techniques help to clear the environment and the body of stagnant or negative energies that may confuse or hinder intentions. Maintaining a clean and tidy physical and energetic space creates a conducive environment for nurturing and cultivating positive intentions.

Example of Guided Meditation and Inner Reflection

Guided Meditation for Intention Clarification

This simple meditation can help clarify your intentions and align your desires with your life path. It can be practiced daily or whenever you feel the need to reconnect with your deeper goals.

Preparation:

- Find a quiet place where you will not be disturbed.

- Sit in a comfortable position, with your back straight and your feet firmly planted on the ground.

- Close your eyes and take a few deep breaths to relax completely.

Phase 1: Calming the Mind

- Begin by focusing on your breath. Feel the air entering and exiting your nostrils.

- With each exhale, let go of tensions and disturbing thoughts.

- Imagine that each thought is like a leaf floating away on a calm river.

Phase 2: Searching for Intention

- Once the mind is calmed, bring your attention to your heart, imagining each breath illuminating it more.

- Ask yourself: "What is my deepest intention in this moment of my life?"

- Let the answer emerge naturally, without forcing it. It may come in the form of words, images, feelings, or a sudden knowing.

Phase 3: Visualization and Refinement

- Once a clear intention emerges, visualize it as a luminous object in your heart, shining and expanding with each breath.

- Now, imagine seeing yourself in the future as you live out this intention. Visualize the details: Where are you? What are you doing? Who is with you?

- See how this intention integrates into your life, noting the positive emotions and feelings of fulfillment that arise from it.

Phase 4: Affirmation and Conclusion

- Affirm to yourself that this is your intention, saying: "I welcome this intention into my life. I am open and ready to manifest it."

- Slowly bring your attention back to the present, gently moving your hands and feet.

- When you feel ready, open your eyes and return to your day, carrying with you the clarity and calmness achieved.

Post-Meditation Tips

After the meditation, it can be helpful to jot down any insights or visualized details. This not only helps to remember the intention but also strengthens your commitment to pursue it. Regular practice of this meditation increases internal awareness and promotes a deeper connection with your authentic goals, guiding you step by step toward their realization.

Example of Practical Positive Affirmations

Positive affirmations are powerful tools for strengthening mindset and maintaining focus on one's intentions and goals. When formulated correctly, affirmations can help transform negative thinking into a more constructive and motivating one, promoting greater confidence and determination. Here are some examples of positive affirmations that you can use daily to support various aspects of your life:

For Personal Growth and Self-Esteem:

1. "I am worthy of love and respect from myself and others."

2. "Every day, in every way, I am becoming better and better."

3. "I am a lifelong learner and embrace new growth opportunities with enthusiasm."

4. "I fully and completely accept myself."

For Professional Success:

1. "I am competent, intelligent, and capable."

2. "Every challenge is an opportunity to enhance my skills."

3. "I am a valuable contributor, and my ideas bring innovation."

4. "I am building a career rich in accomplishments and fulfillment."

For Health and Well-being:

1. "Every day, my body grows stronger and healthier."

2. "I nourish my body with food that energizes and rejuvenates it."

3. "I listen kindly to my body's signals and respect its needs."

4. "Calmness and peace come naturally to me; every breath fills me with serenity."

For Relationships and Social Connection:

1. "I attract healthy, stimulating, and mutually enriching relationships."

2. "I express gratitude and appreciation for the people in my life."

3. "I communicate clearly and empathetically with those around me."

4. "Every interaction is an opportunity for meaningful connections."

For Overcoming Obstacles and Challenges:

1. "I face difficulties with courage and resilience."

2. "I am creative and find innovative solutions to problems."

3. "Every obstacle brings me closer to my ultimate goal."

4. "I am stronger than the challenges I encounter."

How to Use Affirmations:

- **Repeat affirmations in the morning**: Spend a few minutes each morning repeating your affirmations. This sets a positive tone for the rest of the day.

- **Use them as mantras during meditation**: Incorporate affirmations into your meditation practice for an even deeper effect.

- **Write them in a journal**: Writing down affirmations can further reinforce their impact.

- **Set reminders**: Use sticky notes or phone reminders to prompt you to repeat your affirmations throughout the day.

Affirmations are most effective when personalized to fit your specific needs and goals. Feel free to adapt the above expressions to better reflect your personal situation and desires.

Examples of Creative Visualization

Creative visualization is a powerful manifestation technique that involves imagination to achieve one's goals and desires. By creating clear and detailed mental images, you can help your subconscious work towards realizing these goals. Here are some practical examples of how to use creative visualization in different areas of your life:

For Professional Success

Goal: Getting a promotion at work

- **Visualization**: Imagine yourself walking into your boss's office, feeling confidence and calm flowing through you. See yourself discussing your recent achievements and how you've overcome specific challenges. Clearly visualize your boss's approving expression and feel the satisfaction of accepting a new position. Continue by imagining yourself in the new role, handling increased responsibilities with competence and joy.

For Health and Well-being

Goal: Improving physical fitness

- **Visualization**: See yourself waking up energized every morning, wearing your workout clothes, and engaging in physical activity that you love. Feel vibrant and strong as you run, swim, or do yoga. Visualize your body becoming more toned and healthy with each workout session. Feel the pleasure of movement and appreciation for your transforming body.

For Personal Relationships

Goal: Building stronger and more meaningful relationships.

- **Visualization**: Imagine a scene with a close friend or partner in a calm and relaxing environment. Visualize an open and honest conversation, where both of you share deep thoughts and feelings. Feel the empathy and intimacy deepening as you talk. See the two of you laughing together, supporting each other, and building happy memories.

For Personal Growth

Goal: Developing a new skill or hobby.

- **Visualization**: Picture yourself enrolling in and attending classes for a new skill, such as playing a musical instrument, painting, or learning a new language. Visualize yourself eagerly absorbing information during classes and practicing with passion. Project yourself into the future, where you proudly show your work to friends and family, receiving praise and encouragement.

How to Practice Creative Visualization

- **Calm Environment**: Find a quiet place where you won't be disturbed. This can be a silent room or a corner of nature you find relaxing.

- **Deep Breathing**: Before you begin, take a few deep breaths to relax the body and mind.

- **Vivid Details**: Use all five senses to make your visualizations as vivid and detailed as possible. The more you can immerse yourself in the details, the more effective the visualization will be.

- **Regularity**: Practice visualization regularly, ideally once or twice a day, to strengthen mental images and their effectiveness in promoting real changes.

Using these creative visualization techniques can significantly increase your ability to achieve personal and professional goals, improve your health and well-being, enrich your relationships, and promote personal growth.

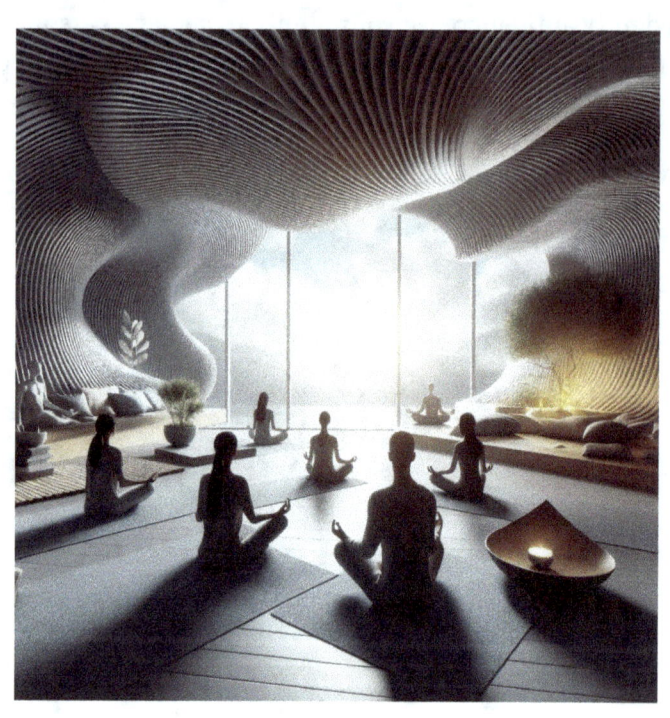

MEDITATION AND VISUALIZATION: OTHER GUIDED PRACTICES TO ESTABLISH A DEEP CONNECTION WITH INTENTION

Meditation and visualization are two powerful practices that can significantly enhance our ability to deeply connect with our intentions. When used together, these techniques not only help clarify and focus our goals but also activate our subconscious to work towards their realization. Here's how these practices can be guided to maximize their potential.

New Meditation and Visualization Techniques for Manifestation

1. Walking Meditation

Walking meditation combines physical movement with mindful attention, ideal for those who find it challenging to sit for long periods.

Guided Practice:

- **Preparation**: Find a quiet path, whether in a park, garden, or even a quiet room where you can walk back and forth.

- **Focus**: Concentrate on your feet as they touch the ground. Feel each step and notice sensations in every part of your foot.

- **Breathing and Steps**: Try to synchronize your breath

with your steps. For example, inhale for four steps and exhale for four steps.

- **Mental Intention**: As you walk, reflect on a specific intention or goal you wish to manifest. Imagine each step physically and spiritually bringing you closer to your goal.

2. Mantra Meditation

Mantras are phrases or sounds repeated during meditation to focus the mind and promote positive vibrations in the body.

Guided Practice:

- **Choose a Mantra**: Select a mantra that resonates with your intention, such as "I am abundance" or "Inner peace."

- **Quiet Environment**: Sit in a calm place and close your eyes. Begin repeating the mantra silently or softly.

- **Concentration and Repetition**: Focus solely on the sound and meaning of the mantra. Repeat it for 10-20 minutes, allowing its vibrations to permeate through your awareness.

- **Visualization with Mantra**: As you repeat the mantra, visualize your intention as already achieved. See yourself living the desired outcome and feel the associated emotions.

3. Creative Visualization with Power Objects

Using physical objects as catalysts for visualization can

strengthen the bond between your intention and tangible manifestation.

Guided Practice:

- **Object Selection**: Choose an object that symbolizes your goal or inspires you, such as a gemstone, piece of jewelry, or natural symbol.

- **Visualization Session**: Hold the object in your hands while closing your eyes. Feel its weight and texture. Begin visualizing your goal as already achieved while holding the object.

- **Emotional Association**: As you hold the object, allow yourself to feel all the positive emotions that come from achieving your goal. Let these sensations intensify with each breath.

- **Daily Use**: Carry the object with you or place it where you can see it every day as a constant visual reminder of your goal.

These techniques offer new ways to integrate meditation and visualization into your daily manifestation practice, helping you establish an even deeper connection with your intentions and manifest your desires more effectively.

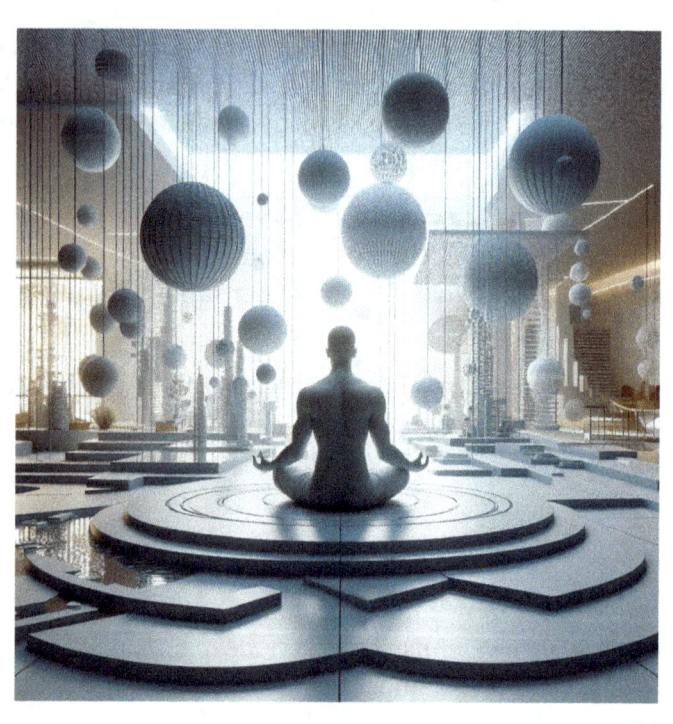

ADDRESSING AND RELEASING ENERGY BLOCKS

In the journey of personal growth and manifestation of one's intentions, addressing and releasing energy blocks is crucial. These blocks can be understood as internal barriers that limit our energy flow, hindering our ability to fully realize our potential. Identifying and overcoming such obstacles requires a deep understanding of internal dynamics and effective techniques to release them.

Identification of Energy Blocks

Energy blocks can manifest in various ways, including recurring negative thought patterns, suppressed emotions such as fear or anger, and even through physical symptoms like muscle tension or chronic discomfort. Identifying them requires careful self-examination through various techniques:

1. **Mindful Self-Observation:**

Mindfulness and meditation can help become more aware of your thoughts and emotions. Dedicate time each day to meditation allows you to observe the habitual patterns of your thinking and emotional reactions that may indicate the presence of energy blocks.

2. **Emotional Journaling**:

Keeping a journal of your emotions and thoughts can

reveal recurring patterns or themes that may be symptomatic of deeper blocks. Writing about how you feel in relation to various aspects of your life can help you identify areas of stagnation or resistance.

3. Body Feedback:

The body often tracks psychological tensions in the form of physical pain or discomfort. Techniques such as yoga, tai chi, or simply stretching can help recognize where the body feels stuck or rigid, providing clues to related energy blocks.

Overcoming Energy Blocks

Once identified, the next step is to actively work on releasing them. This can be done through various practices that help release trapped energy and promote a more harmonious energy flow:

1. Emotional Release Techniques:

Methods such as Emotional Freedom Technique (EFT), which involves tapping on specific energy points of the body while focusing on specific emotions or memories, can be extremely effective in releasing energy blocks related to old emotions.

2. Energy Work:

Practices like Reiki, pranic healing, or other forms of

energy therapy can help rebalance the body's energy, facilitating the release of blocks and promoting a state of overall well-being.

3. **Psychotherapy and Counseling**:

For particularly persistent or complex blocks, working with a therapist can be helpful. Therapy can offer significant insights and tools to address and release entrenched emotional and cognitive patterns.

4. **Visualization and Affirmations**:

Using visualization to imagine the flow of energy releasing from blocks can be enhanced by using positive affirmations that support release and healing.

Conclusion

Addressing and releasing energy blocks is an ongoing process that can significantly improve the quality of life and increase your ability to manifest your desires. Through self-awareness, energy work, and therapeutic support, it is possible to break free from the chains of old patterns and pave the way for a freer and more fulfilled existence.

TOOLS AND TECHNIQUES FOR MANIFESTATION

Using speech and thought for manifestation

The art of manifestation is based on the idea that words and thoughts are not mere expressions or internal reflections but powerful tools that can shape reality. When properly directed, words and thoughts can actually create tangible conditions and results in a person's life. This chapter explores how to consciously use speech and thought to influence and manifest concrete desires and goals.

The Power of Conscious Thought

The power of conscious thought is an essential component for anyone aspiring to master the art of manifestation. Thoughts, incessant companions of our existence, manifest both during waking hours and in dreams, influencing not only our internal state but also the external world in often underestimated ways. Contrary to what one might think, thoughts are not mere passages of information; they are rather charged with energy that can shape, distort, create, or destroy the physical reality around us.

This continuous mental activity can have a significant impact on our lives if not properly managed. Without conscious direction, thoughts can wander into negative or destructive territories, creating scenarios of anxiety, fear, and uncertainty that may manifest in undesirable outcomes. Therefore, learning to govern thoughts through awareness is a crucial step towards effectively manifesting one's desires and goals.

The practice of conscious thought begins with careful observation and acknowledgment of one's mental patterns. This involves the ability to notice thoughts as soon as they arise, understand their origins and emotional impact, and consciously choose which ones to cultivate and which ones to release. For example, when a negative or limiting thought arises, instead of getting caught up in the vortex of automatic reactivity, one can consciously choose to replace it with a more positive and constructive thought.

Furthermore, the practice can be enriched through techniques such as mindfulness meditation, which helps center the mind and reduce the chaotic flow of thoughts. This type of meditation not only calms the mind but also hones the ability to focus on specific intentions without being distracted by irrelevant thoughts. As this practice deepens, it becomes possible to maintain clarity of intent even in daily activities, making every thought a proactive step towards achieving personal goals.

Learning to use conscious thought means transforming an automatic mental function into a powerful tool of creation and manifestation. Through awareness and active management of thoughts, new possibilities for personal growth and fulfillment can be opened, demonstrating that the mind, when properly directed, is one of the most powerful tools at our disposal for shaping reality in our favor.

1. **Awareness and Intentionality:**

The first step in mastering thought for manifestation is to be fully aware of one's thoughts. This requires a mindful observer who notices when the mind deviates towards unproductive or negative thoughts and gently redirects it towards more positive and constructive ones.

2. **Thinking Constructively**:

It is essential to cultivate a way of thinking that is inherently positive and solution-oriented rather than problem-focused. This involves training the mind to see possibilities and opportunities in every situation rather than obstacles or barriers.

The Power of Articulated Words

Words are physical manifestations of thought and have the power to alter reality in ways that thought alone cannot. Speaking words, whether affirmations, speeches, or dialogues, can solidify thought and begin to manifest it in the external world.

1. **Positive Affirmations:**

Affirmations are positively formulated statements that are repeated regularly to reinforce a vision or intention. For example, repeating daily "I am abundant and attract wealth in every form" can help internalize this reality and manifest it.

2. **Speaking with Intent**:

Every word you speak should be considered for its potential impact. This means avoiding negative or self-limiting speech and focusing on words that express your intention for success, happiness, health, and abundance.

Guided Visualization to Reinforce Thought and Word

Combining thought and word in a guided visualization practice can amplify their power of manifestation:

1. **Creating a Detailed Mental Scenario**:

Dedicate time each day to vividly visualize your goals as already achieved. Imagine living the life you desire, feeling the emotions associated with that reality, and seeing yourself actively participating in that life.

2. **Incorporating Speech into the Visual Process:**

As you visualize, speak aloud or mentally the words that describe that scenario. Use language that reinforces the achievement of goals, as if narrating a story that has already happened.

Conclusion

The conscious use of speech and thought for manifestation is not just a spiritual or metaphysical practice; it is a skill that can be developed and refined to significantly improve the quality of one's life. Through awareness, self-control, and regular practice, every individual has the power to transform their thoughts and words into effective tools for personal realization and the creation of a desired reality.

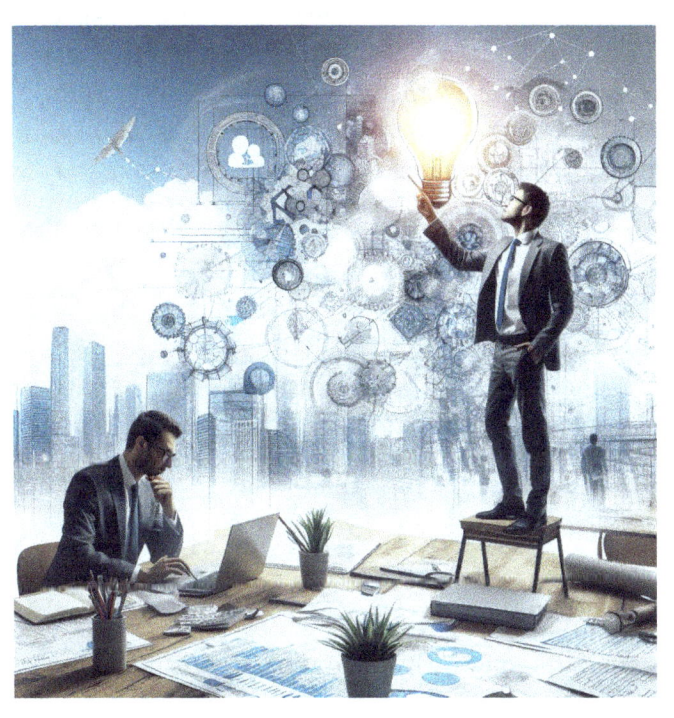

CREATING A DAILY ROUTINE

TIPS FOR INTEGRATING MANIFESTATION INTO EVERYDAY LIFE

Integrating the practice of manifestation into everyday life requires a systematic and intentional approach. Creating a daily routine helps establish consistency and maximize the effectiveness of manifestation techniques. Here are some detailed steps and tips for building a daily routine that facilitates personal realization and the transformation of desires into concrete reality.

Establishing a Fixed Schedule

An effective routine begins with dedicating specific moments of the day to manifestation practice. This helps create a habit and ensures that practices are not overlooked.

1. **Morning**:

Start the day with meditation or positive affirmations. The morning is an ideal time to set intentions for the day, as the mind is still fresh and relatively free from the distractions of the day.

2. **Afternoon**:

Dedicate a few minutes in the afternoon to a brief reflection session or adjustment of your intentions. This can serve as a reminder of your aspirations and as a check to stay on course during the day.

3. **Evening**:

Before going to bed, practice visualization. This is the time to relax and "program" the subconscious with images of the desired future. The evening is also a great time to keep a gratitude journal, noting what you have achieved or steps taken towards your goals.

Creating a Supportive Environment

The environment in which you live and work can significantly influence your ability to manifest effectively.

1. **Personal Space**:

Maintain a corner of your home dedicated to your manifestation practices. This space should be neat, quiet, and inspiring. You can decorate it with objects symbolizing your goals, such as pictures of places you want to visit or items representing success.

2. **Supportive Materials**:

Use tools that help focus your attention and enhance your practice, such as candles, incense, crystals, or relaxing music. These elements can help create a relaxing and motivating atmosphere.

Consistency and Flexibility

While consistency is key to building and maintaining the habit of manifestation, it's also important to remain flexible. Life can be unpredictable, and your routine should have enough room to adapt to unexpected circumstances.

1. **Adaptability**:

If for some reason you're unable to follow your routine, don't get discouraged. Adapt the practices to the available time or specific context. Even a few minutes of meditation or affirmations can be powerful.

2. **Regular Evaluation**:

Periodically review your routine to ensure it remains aligned with your current goals and that you continue to find pleasure and value in the practices you're performing. Modify activities if necessary to keep your practice fresh.

Conclusion

Building a daily routine for manifestation will not only help you achieve your goals but also live a more intentional and fulfilling life. This routine transforms manifestation practices from activities you might occasionally do into fundamental components of your lifestyle, ensuring that your daily actions are aligned with your deepest desires.

JOURNALING AND PROGRESS TRACKING

THE IMPORTANCE OF DOCUMENTING JOURNEYS AND ACHIEVEMENTS

Journaling and progress tracking are essential tools in the personal manifestation process. Systematically documenting your journeys, achievements, and even failures can have a profound impact on your ability to achieve your goals. These practices not only provide a tangible overview of progress but also help maintain motivation, reflect on behaviors, and clarify thoughts and emotions.

Importance of Journaling

Journaling is a transformative art that goes beyond the traditional concept of a personal diary of daily events. It is a powerful and reflective tool that allows individuals to shape, voice, and structure the complex flows of their thoughts and emotions. Through the practice of journaling, fleeting thoughts and feelings, often ephemeral and difficult to grasp, are not only captured but also examined and understood more deeply.

This process of crystallizing thoughts is vital for several reasons. Firstly, it helps organize information and emotions that might otherwise remain confused or overlapping. Writing down thoughts allows one to distance oneself from them, offering a more objective perspective. This detachment enables clearer evaluation and can facilitate better emotional management, especially in times of stress or change.

Moreover, journaling functions as a mechanism for self-explanation, where the simple act of writing helps clarify and define problems, ideas, and aspirations. This can be particularly useful in times of decision-making or transition, allowing one to discover what is truly valued and which steps to take forward. Writing can also reveal recurring patterns of behavior and thought, facilitating the identification of any personal obstacles or barriers to growth or goal achievement.

Regular journaling practice can also increase self-awareness and promote continuous improvement. Putting successes and failures into writing helps build a coherent life narrative and strengthen personal identity. With a greater understanding of oneself, it is possible to navigate life with greater confidence and purpose, guiding actions and decisions towards goals that truly reflect one's values and desires.

Finally, journaling offers a safe haven for free and private expression, a place where ideas and feelings can be explored without judgment. This space for reflection can become a source of great comfort and support, a silent yet powerful companion in managing life's daily challenges.

In summary, journaling is much more than a simple record of events; it is a dynamic process of self-exploration and understanding that can significantly enhance mental clarity, emotional balance, and personal direction. Through constant journaling practice, it is possible to transform the internal whirlwind of thoughts and emotions into a clear and deliberate path towards achieving personal goals and aspirations.

1. Mental Clarity and Focus:

Regularly jotting down your thoughts, feelings, successes, and challenges in journaling is a powerful tool for self-awareness and mental organization. This method not only facilitates better management of emotions and daily experiences but also provides a crucial means of maintaining a clear and focused mind. Through journaling, you can articulate not only what you are experiencing in the present but also actively shape the future direction of your actions.

The process of writing helps decompress complex thoughts and turn them into something tangible and manageable. This can be particularly helpful in times of confusion or emotional overload when thoughts seem to overlap and it becomes difficult to maintain focus. Putting these thoughts and feelings on paper allows you to see them more clearly, recognize patterns or recurring issues, and address them more systematically.

In addition to improving emotional management, journaling hones the ability to set and maintain goals. With a clear view of your own mental states and recorded emotional reactions over time, it is easier to outline realistic and achievable goals. Journaling thus becomes a map guiding the individual through the complex terrain of daily life, indicating both obstacles overcome and milestones yet to be reached.

Furthermore, documenting successes and challenges serves as continuous feedback on your life path. Each journal entry can serve as a moment of reflection, a checkpoint to assess whether the actions taken are aligned with long-term intentions. This practice can be incredibly rewarding, offering the opportunity to celebrate successes, learn from mistakes, and, if necessary, readjust plans for the future.

In summary, the mental clarity and focus achieved through journaling are indispensable for anyone wishing to live an intentional and targeted life. Regularly writing about your thoughts and experiences not only helps keep the mind clear and organized but also provides essential support for effectively navigating towards your goals. With each written page, you refine your ability to better understand yourself and to move consciously in the world.

2. **Recognition of Patterns:**

Rereading old writings can reveal patterns or trends in your behavior, thinking, or emotions that you may not otherwise notice. Identifying these patterns is crucial for making conscious changes in your life.

3. **Evaluation and Repositioning**:

Journaling offers an opportunity to periodically evaluate progress towards your goals. If you find yourself off track, you can reposition and adjust your plans accordingly.

Progress Tracking

Progress tracking goes hand in hand with journaling.

While journaling may include more descriptive and reflective details, progress tracking is often more structured and quantitative.

1. **Setting Measurable Indicators**:

Establish clear and measurable performance indicators for your goals. This may include specific numbers, deadlines, or completed milestones. Tracking these indicators allows you to see how far you have progressed and how much more you need to do to reach your ultimate goal.

2. **Using Tracking Tools**:

Utilize tools such as habit tracking apps, spreadsheets, or physical planners to keep order in your tracking process. These tools can help you stay organized and keep your focus.

3. **Celebrating Successes**:

Documenting and celebrating small successes along the way is vital. This not only boosts your self-esteem and motivation but also strengthens your belief in your ability to manifest your desires.

Integration of Journaling and Tracking into Daily Routine

To derive the maximum benefit from these practices,

integrate them into your daily life:

- Dedicate Daily Time:

Set aside a specific time each day, perhaps in the morning for planning and in the evening for reflection and documentation.

- Make the Practice Enjoyable:

Use a beautiful notebook for your journal or a thoughtfully designed app for progress tracking, making the practice aesthetically pleasing and personally meaningful.

- Periodic Reflection:

Every month, conduct a broader review of your progress, evaluating what has worked, what hasn't, and how you can further improve.

In conclusion, journaling and progress tracking are not only fundamental to goal achievement but also to personal development and self-awareness. These practices, implemented with consistency and introspection, can transform manifestation from a mere desire into a tangible and measurable reality.

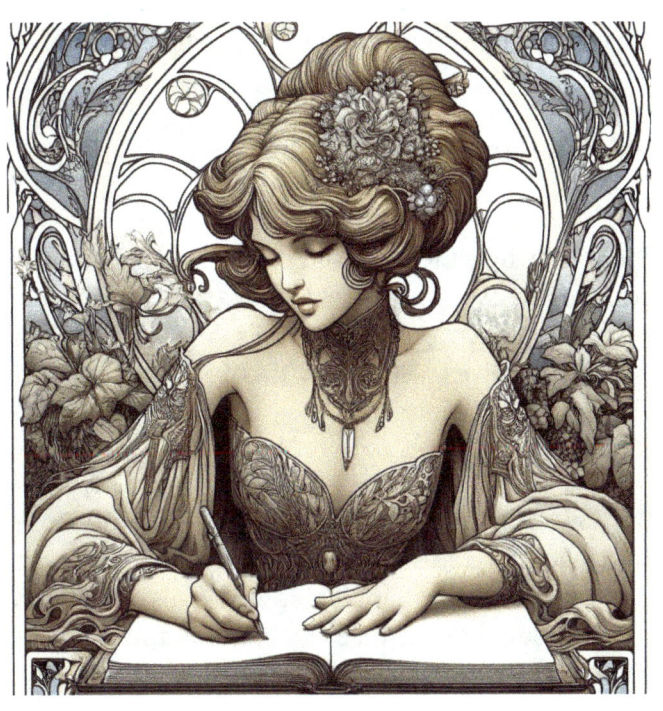

STORIES OF SUCCESS

In this chapter, we explore four evocative stories of individuals who have transformed their lives through the application of Dolores Cannon's methods. These narratives not only celebrate successes but also offer profound insights into the mechanisms behind these changes, providing a window into human potential and the power of healing and personal transformation.

Story 1: Elena's Renaissance

Background: Elena, a successful lawyer, found herself drained by excessive stress and a life lacking personal meaning. Discovering Cannon's methods led her to explore past lives, where she discovered she was a painter in the Italian Renaissance.

Experience: Using QHHT, Elena relived moments from her past life, rediscovering a lost passion for art that awakened her dormant creativity. This revelation gave her the courage to reduce her hours in the legal field and pursue a new career as an artist.

Lesson: Elena's story demonstrates how understanding past lives can unlock hidden potential and inspire radical changes in career and personal passions.

Story 2: Giorgio's Healing

Background: Giorgio, a war veteran, suffered from chronic PTSD that did not improve with conventional treatments. Through QHHT, he discovered that his trauma was connected not only to recent experiences but also to a past life as a soldier in World War I.

Experience: In his sessions, Giorgio confronted and reprocessed the traumatic experiences of both lives, leading to a significant reduction in his PTSD symptoms.

Lesson: Giorgio's healing reveals how Cannon's methods can facilitate profound emotional healing, addressing the roots of trauma that may extend beyond current existence.

Story 3: Aisha's Spiritual Transformation

Background: Aisha, a computer engineer, felt increasingly disillusioned by the lack of purpose in her life. Through QHHT sessions, she discovered deep spiritual connections and inner guidance she had never considered before.

Experience: Aisha began integrating spiritual practices into her daily life and found a new sense of peace and direction, eventually becoming a spiritual guide for others.

Lesson: This story highlights how exploring past lives

and connecting with the Higher Self can open new paths for meaning and personal satisfaction.

Story 4: James's Awakening

Background: James, a failed entrepreneur, was facing bankruptcy and depression. Through the discovery of Cannon's methods, he explored unrealized potentials in past lives that inspired him to rethink his approaches in business.

Experience: Visualization and affirmation, integrated into his daily routine, helped James rebuild his career with a new vision based on creativity and innovation, leading him to found a successful startup in the technology sector.

Lesson: James's transformation demonstrates how Cannon's techniques can be used not only for personal healing but also for professional success and recovery from seemingly devastating failures.

Story 5: Clara, Rediscovering Self-Esteem

Background: Clara, a 28-year-old woman, worked in a small marketing company. Despite professional success, she struggled with self-esteem issues and difficult personal relationships, often feeling inadequate and dissatisfied with her personal life.

Experience: After reading about Dolores Cannon's techniques, Clara decided to explore past life regression, hoping to find a radical explanation for her insecurities. During her first QHHT session, Clara discovered she was a talented painter in France in the 18th century, but whose work was constantly discredited and minimized by her male contemporaries.

Impact: Revealing this past life was a turning point for Clara. Understanding that the origins of her low self-esteem could be traced back to a previous life, where she was not properly valued, allowed her to recognize that her feelings of inadequacy were not inherently tied to her true identity.

Techniques Used: After the session, Clara began a journey of positive affirmations and guided visualizations, focusing on images of herself receiving recognition and appreciation for her creative work. Every morning, she devoted time to visualizing her personal art exhibition, where visitors praised her art and where she felt proud and confident in her abilities.

Results: Over time, Clara's self-esteem significantly improved. She began to value her work and ideas more, not only in her career but also in her personal relationships. This newfound confidence allowed her to advance to positions of greater responsibility in her work and to build healthier and more reciprocal relationships.

Lesson: Clara's story illustrates the importance of addressing and reprocessing past wounds, whether they come from this life or past lives. Her experiences demonstrate how past life regression and visualization can be powerful tools for overcoming deep emotional blocks and promoting profound personal change.

This story is an example of how recognizing and reprocessing past experiences can free an individual from cycles of self-doubt and insecurity, allowing for deep and lasting transformation. Clara represents many of us who carry invisible burdens, and her story offers hope and inspiration for those seeking to find and use their own voice and value in the world.

These stories represent only a small fraction of the infinite possibilities offered by Dolores Cannon's methods. Each case study offers valuable insight into how past, present, and future can interweave in surprising ways, guiding individuals from all walks of life towards a more fulfilling and realized life.

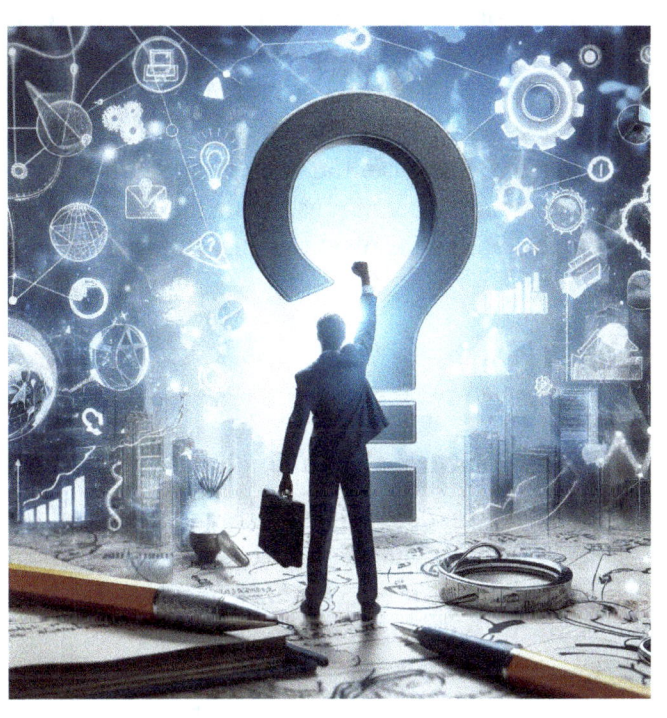

ANALYSIS OF WHAT WORKED AND WHAT DIDN'T

LESSONS LEARNED FROM CASE STUDIES

From the thorough examination of success stories resulting from the application of Dolores Cannon's methods, we can draw important lessons on the factors that positively contributed to the outcomes, as well as on aspects that posed challenges. Analyzing what worked and what didn't is essential to fully understand how past life regression techniques can be optimized and personalized to better meet the needs of individuals.

What Worked

1. **Personalization of Approach**:

Personalization of approach emerged as one of the most crucial aspects in success stories related to the use of Dolores Cannon's techniques. The practice of meticulously tailoring therapy strategies to individual specificities has been shown not only effective but essential in facilitating profound and lasting transformations in clients' lives.

Personalization goes beyond simply tweaking techniques to fit different people. It involves a careful assessment of personal experiences, emotional blocks, cultural contexts, and even psychological predispositions. This process typically begins with a series of in-depth interviews or questionnaires that help the therapist understand the client's life history, current challenges, and future goals.

For example, in the case of someone coping with loss or grief, the therapist might incorporate specific grief support techniques into past life regression, ensuring the session is directed at healing deep emotional wounds. Alternatively, for someone seeking to overcome creative blocks, the approach may focus on releasing limiting beliefs and exploring past lives where the client lived as an artist or creative.

Personalization requires active collaboration between the client and the therapist. Together, they must explore different dimensions of the client's life to uncover areas that need greater attention. This synergy enables the therapist to create a therapeutic path that is not only targeted but also dynamically adaptable to the client's reactions and evolutions during the process.

The use of customized techniques and tools is fundamental in this process. This may include using specific types of visualization, tailoring the language of affirmations to resonate more deeply with the client's individual experience, or selecting particular stories or metaphors during regression sessions that echo the client's personal life.

Another critical aspect of personalization is the ongoing monitoring and adaptation of techniques used. Each session offers new insights and information that can guide further personalizations. This iterative approach ensures that the treatment remains relevant and impactful for the client, adapting to their changing needs and discoveries along the healing journey.

Personalizing the approach not only significantly increases the effectiveness of manifestation and healing techniques but also strengthens the trust relationship between client and therapist. By recognizing and honoring each individual's uniqueness, the therapist can facilitate a transformation journey that is as unique as the person themselves. This methodology deeply respects the complexity of human experience and confirms that the path to healing and personal realization is as personal as it is universal.

2. **Continual Support**:

Continual support after regression sessions emerges as a fundamental pillar in the success of manifestation and personal healing practices. Commitment to providing ongoing support to clients has been shown essential in consolidating the benefits of initial sessions and promoting sustainable change over time. This form of post-session support includes various elements that together create a care and growth ecosystem that transcends the individual therapy experience.

1. **Regular Follow-ups**:

Regular follow-up sessions are crucial to ensure that clients stay on track towards their long-term goals. These meetings allow addressing any new challenges that emerge as the client integrates insights and transformations experienced during regression. They also offer the opportunity to reinforce coping strategies and reaffirm the client's personal and spiritual goals.

2. **Self-Help Resources**:

Providing clients with access to a variety of self-help

resources can significantly empower their healing journey. This may include guided meditations that help maintain calm and centeredness, books and articles that delve into the theoretical aspects of the techniques used, or online videos and workshops to promote understanding and application of self-healing practices.

3. **Support Groups**:

Participation in support groups or practice communities can provide an additional level of emotional and practical support. Sharing experiences with others going through similar paths can not only alleviate the sense of isolation but also inspire and motivate participants to continue their personal work. Support groups offer a platform for the exchange of stories, strategies, and mutual encouragement.

4. **Ongoing Counscling**:

The availability of ongoing counseling, whether psychological, spiritual, or practical, is another essential element of continual support. Having access to professionals who can offer guidance and advice allows clients to navigate the complexities of their transformations with greater confidence.

The long-term impact of continual support is evident in the stories of those who have experienced substantial improvements in their emotional, mental, and physical well-being. Continual support helps integrate changes at a deep level, making the effects of regression sessions enduring. Additionally, it establishes a safety net that can accelerate healing and foster ongoing personal growth.

In summary, continual support is an irreplaceable aspect of an effective therapeutic approach in the field of past life regression and manifestation practices. By ensuring constant commitment and a wide range of supportive resources, it can be ensured that transformations initiated in sessions have a positive and lasting impact, guiding individuals towards a more fulfilling and realized life. This type of support demonstrates a commitment to the holistic care of the client, recognizing that the journey of healing and transformation is often long and requires a dedication that goes beyond the initial sessions.

3. **Integration with Other Well-Being Practices**:

The most positive stories were those in which past life regression was integrated with other well-being practices, such as meditation, yoga, and cognitive-behavioral therapy. This holistic approach helped individuals better manage their discoveries and apply the lessons learned more effectively and harmoniously in their daily lives.

What Didn't Work

1. **Unrealistic Expectations**:

One of the most common obstacles was the emergence of unrealistic expectations. Some individuals expected past life regression to immediately solve complex issues without further personal efforts or changes in their lifestyle. This sometimes led to disappointments and reduced effectiveness of the treatment.

2. Lack of Follow-Up:

Another issue encountered was the lack of adequate follow-up after initial sessions. Without continual support, some people found it difficult to maintain necessary changes or properly interpret their experiences and insights.

3. Resistance to Change:

In some cases, significant resistance to change emerged. Regardless of the insights gained during sessions, some individuals struggled to accept or integrate these learnings into their lives, often due to fear, entrenched habits, or lack of a supportive environment.

Lessons Learned

From these analyses, it is clear that the key to success in past life regression techniques lies not only in the methodology itself but also in how it is implemented and followed over time. The following lessons can be drawn to enhance the future effectiveness of these practices:

- **Setting Clear Expectations:** It is crucial for therapists to help clients set realistic expectations before starting treatment.
- **Holistic and Continual Support**: Providing continual support and integrating other well-being practices can significantly increase the effectiveness of the healing and personal growth process.

- **Personalization and Adaptability**: Tailoring techniques to individual needs and being ready to modify the approach based on the client's response are crucial for achieving the best possible results.

By learning from these successes and failures, we can continue to refine and enrich manifestation and personal transformation practices, making the healing and growth process accessible and fruitful for an even greater number of people.

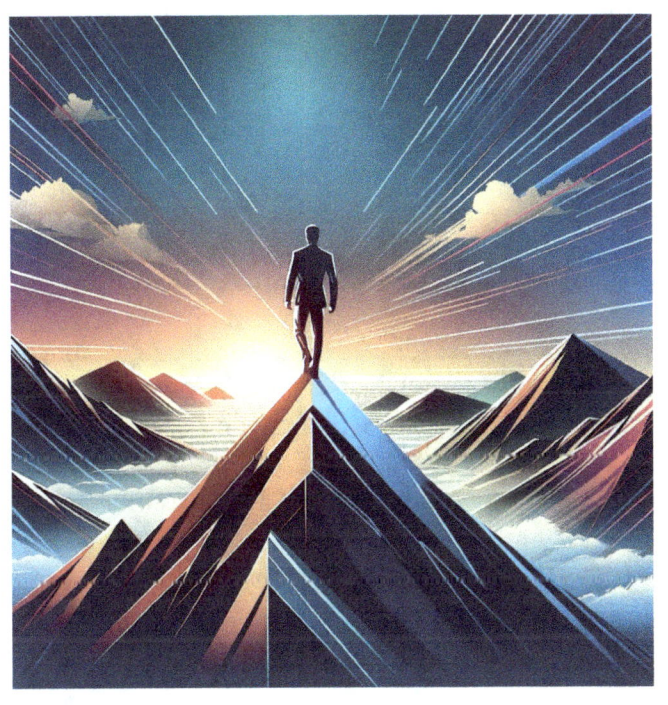

OVERCOMING CHALLENGES

COMMON CHALLENGES IN MANIFESTATION

The road to manifestation is often winding and fraught with challenges that may seem insurmountable. However, understanding and overcoming these difficulties is essential for personal progress and the realization of one's desires. In this chapter, we will explore the common challenges associated with manifestation, providing insights and strategies for effectively addressing them.

Common Challenges in Manifestation

Manifestation is not just a process of positive thinking and waiting for things to happen. It is an active and dynamic journey that requires commitment, patience, and a deep understanding of the laws that govern the universe and human interaction with it. Below are some of the most common challenges that people encounter during this journey.

1. **Doubt and Skepticism:**

One of the greatest challenges in manifestation is overcoming internal doubt and skepticism, feelings that can erect significant barriers on the path to realizing one's desires. These energetic obstacles are not merely emotional; they deeply influence the ability to attract and create the reality one desires. Often, doubt and skepticism root themselves in the fear of the unknown, a nearly universal human condition that makes us fear what we cannot predict or control. Additionally, the perception of not having control over future events or outcomes can intensify these feelings, making individuals feel powerless in the face of life's forces.

Past experiences also play a crucial role in this context. Past disappointments or failures can leave a lasting imprint, leading people to doubt their abilities and the value of their efforts. This skepticism can be particularly paralyzing when attempting to adopt new paths or reinvent oneself in ways that require confidence not only in one's abilities but also in the manifestation process itself.

The challenge, then, is not only to recognize and understand the origin of these doubts but also to develop effective strategies to mitigate or overcome them. This process can begin with self-reflection and acknowledgment that doubt and skepticism, while understandable responses, do not necessarily have to define the course of future actions. The key lies in rebuilding confidence through small successes and constant reaffirmation of one's intentions and goals. Additionally, practices such as meditation, positive affirmation, and visualization can help recalibrate the mind toward a more open and receptive attitude, essential for breaking down the barriers of doubt and advancing with greater confidence and determination toward the realization of one's dreams.

Ultimately, overcoming doubt and skepticism requires active and continuous commitment, not only to change thought patterns but also to create an internal environment that supports personal growth and transformation. With a conscious and deliberate approach, it is possible to transform uncertainty and fear into allies that inform but do not hinder the path to manifestation.

2. **Impatience and Unrealistic Expectations**:

Impatience and unrealistic expectations pose a significant challenge in the manifestation process, particularly in an era dominated by the culture of instant gratification. Our modern society often emphasizes quick results and instant success, profoundly influencing our perception of time and personal achievement. This predisposition can create considerable tension when engaging in the manifestation process, which by its nature requires patience and an understanding that each desire materializes according to its own intrinsic timeline, often independent of our immediate will.

When expected results do not materialize within the hoped-for time frame, impatience can quickly turn into frustration and disillusionment. This state of mind is not only counterproductive but can also disrupt the energetic flow necessary to attract what we desire. The key to managing this challenge is not so much in trying to speed up results to appease our impatience, but rather in recalibrating our expectations and cultivating a more patient and realistic perspective.

Overcoming impatience requires a fundamental shift in the perception of time and the process. It is helpful to adopt practices such as meditation or mindfulness techniques, which help center the mind and reduce anxiety related to waiting. These techniques can also increase our awareness of the present moment, reducing the tendency to focus excessively on the future and desired outcomes. Additionally, it is beneficial to set short-term goals that can be more easily achieved and lead to incremental satisfactions, thereby maintaining enthusiasm and a sense of progress.

Another crucial aspect is the acceptance that the journey toward realizing grand ambitions is often marked by small progressive steps rather than giant leaps. Celebrating these small successes can alleviate feelings of stagnation and strengthen confidence in the long-term manifestation process. Finally, it is essential to periodically review and, if necessary, adjust our expectations to keep them aligned with the reality of our unique personal journey.

In summary, managing impatience and realigning unrealistic expectations not only enhances our ability to manifest successfully but also enriches the life experience, teaching us the value of perseverance, resilience, and the recognition that anything worth having deserves time and dedication.

3. **Lack of Clarity**:

Having fuzzy goals or unclear intentions is another common challenge. Without a precise vision of what one wants to achieve, the universe cannot respond clearly and precisely. Lack of clarity can therefore lead to confused outcomes or ones that are not fully aligned with the individual's desires.

4. **Incongruence between Intentions and Actions:**

An additional challenge arises when there is a disconnect between what a person wishes to manifest and the actions they take. For example, aspiring to serenity while perpetuating interpersonal conflicts can hinder the achievement of that desired inner peace.

5. External Influences and Negative Environment:

The surrounding environment and external influences play a crucial role in the manifestation process, either facilitating or hindering the achievement of our goals. The nature of our everyday environment, from the people we interact with to the atmospheres we frequent, can have a significant impact on our energy, mood, and ability to focus and pursue our deepest desires.

Negative individuals, for example, can heavily influence our approach to life and our dreams. Regular interactions with individuals who express skepticism, cynicism, or simply a worldview inclined toward pessimism can erode our positivity and diminish our motivation. This type of negative energy can introduce doubt and insecurity, making us less inclined to pursue our goals with the boldness and determination required.

Similarly, chaotic or disorderly spaces can reflect and reinforce a sense of internal confusion and mental disorganization. A cluttered physical environment not only distracts attention but can also symbolize and perpetuate a state of internal disorder, making it more challenging to maintain a clear and focused vision of our manifestation goals. External chaos can easily translate into internal chaos, which in turn can hinder the process of clarifying our intentions and personal realization.

Furthermore, a cultural climate of pessimism, whether within a social group, a work environment, or a broader community, can negatively influence our worldview and personal expectations. When immersed in a context that constantly emphasizes limitations and obstacles rather than opportunities and potentialities, we may become less inclined to believe in the possibility of changing our reality and in the personal power of manifestation.

Faced with these environmental challenges, it is essential for manifestation practitioners to actively seek to build and maintain a supportive environment. This may involve practical changes such as reorganizing living and working spaces to create order and harmony, intentionally surrounding oneself with positive and inspiring people, and engaging in communities that share an optimistic and progressive outlook on life. Promoting an environment that supports personal growth and positivity can greatly enhance the ability to manifest one's desires, transforming spaces and relationships into resources rather than obstacles on the path to personal realization.

Strategies for Overcoming Challenges

For every challenge, there are strategies that can help overcome them, strengthening the path to manifestation.

1. **Strengthening Faith and Patience:**

The practice of meditation and participation in support groups or communities of thought can strengthen faith in one's manifestation abilities and help maintain patience during the process.

2. Defining Clear Goals:

Using techniques such as vision boarding or journaling can help clarify goals and detail the specific steps necessary to achieve them. Clarity of goals is crucial for directing energies correctly.

3. Aligning Actions and Intentions:

It is crucial that daily actions are in line with manifestation intentions. This may require regular self-examination and adaptation of habits to ensure they actively support desires and goals.

4. Cultivating a Positive Environment:

Modifying the environment to make it more supportive can have a significant impact. This may involve reducing interactions with negative individuals, improving the physical organization of living or working space, and immersing oneself in literature and media that reinforce a positive outlook and infinite possibilities.

Through identifying and understanding the common challenges in manifestation and applying targeted strategies to overcome them, it is possible not only to address these obstacles but also to use them as springboards for further personal growth and realization. Overcoming these challenges not only accelerates the manifestation process but also enriches the journey, making it a deeply gratifying experience of learning and transformation.

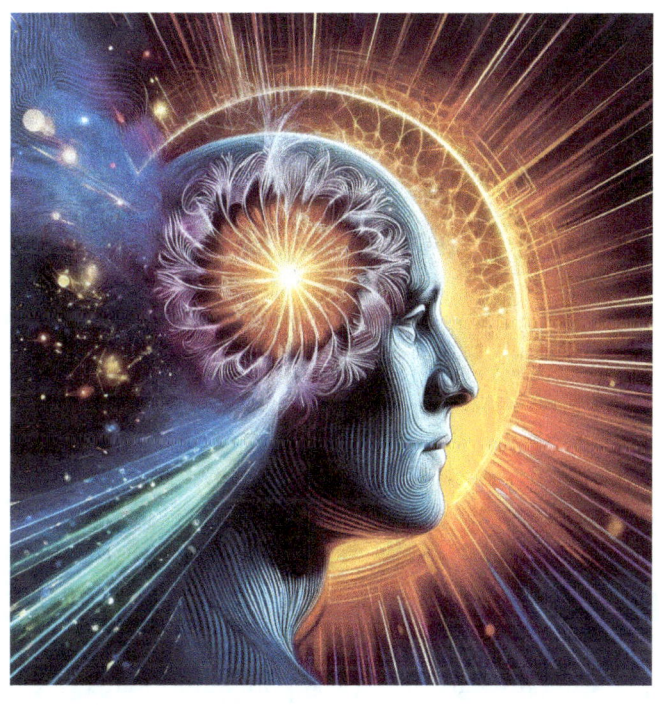

MAINTAINING MOTIVATION

Maintaining motivation over time, especially when desired results are slow to manifest, is a crucial challenge in the manifestation process. Motivation is the fuel that drives us to continue our commitment to our goals despite difficulties or delays. Below, we will explore various practical and psychological strategies to keep motivation high and effectively manage periods of apparent stagnation or slowness in achieving results.

Recognizing and Celebrating Small Successes

An effective method to maintain motivation during the long and sometimes arduous manifestation process is to recognize and celebrate every progress made, regardless of its size. This practice is particularly useful because it allows us to concretely visualize movement towards the ultimate goal, transforming the journey into a series of small successes that can be easily observed and measured. Celebrating progress, even those that may seem insignificant or minor, plays a crucial role in reinforcing the perception that every action, decision, and small step taken is indeed a step forward towards the desired goal.

Incorporating into the manifestation process the practice of setting intermediate goals is an additional strategy that amplifies this effect. These goals serve as milestones along the way, offering regular checkpoints that not only allow progress to be assessed but also celebrated. These moments of reflection and celebration can provide a renewed sense of purpose and a boost of motivational energy, especially when the journey becomes more challenging and the final destination may still seem far away.

The act of celebrating these small successes is essential for maintaining a positive and proactive attitude. This includes, for example, taking a moment to reflect on the day's achievements, writing about progress in one's journal, or sharing victories with friends or colleagues who support personal efforts. Each celebration serves to remind the individual of the value of their commitment and the importance of continuing to pursue their goals with dedication.

This methodology not only helps maintain motivation but also encourages a mindset of continuous growth, where every step forward, no matter how small, is a building block upon the previous one. This creates a chain of successes that, step by step, inevitably leads to the achievement of long-term goals. In summary, recognizing and celebrating every progress, and setting intermediate goals along the way, are practices that not only keep motivation high but also strengthen confidence in one's ability to manifest any desired intention.

Setting Clear and Measurable Goals

Clarity of goals is a fundamental pillar for maintaining motivation along the path to personal and professional realization. Well-defined, specific, and measurable goals create a clear direction and a quantifiable path that facilitates progress monitoring and performance evaluation. This aspect is crucial because without a clear goal, efforts can become scattered and less effective, diluting motivation and reducing the likelihood of achieving desired results.

The adoption of the SMART methodology (Specific, Measurable, Achievable, Relevant, Time-bound) is particularly useful in this context. "Specific" goals allow focusing on what is essential, avoiding ambiguities that can lead to confusion or misinterpretation of the goal. Being "Measurable" means that progress towards the goal can be concretely tracked, providing continuous feedback that is vital for adapting strategies and maintaining enthusiasm. Goals should also be "Achievable," that is, realistic and attainable; setting overly ambitious goals can result in frustration and demotivation, while realistic goals promote confidence and determination.

Furthermore, it is important that goals are "Relevant," meaning closely linked to interests, values, and the overall direction one wants to give to their life or career. Aligning goals with personal passions and core values increases emotional investment and intrinsic motivation. Finally, being "Time-bound" implies having a clear deadline, an aspect that instills a sense of urgency and can accelerate action.

The SMART methodology not only helps define goals effectively but also provides a framework through which action can be organized and planned systematically and coherently. This structuring helps maintain motivation even in moments of apparent stagnation or when results are slow to manifest because every small step taken is a step closer to the final goal. By using this methodology, individuals can visualize the overall path and every intermediate success, reinforcing confidence in their abilities and determination to continue despite difficulties.

In conclusion, the importance of clear and well-structured goals cannot be underestimated in the manifestation process. They not only direct action but are also a source of continuous motivation, facilitating a journey to success that is as effective as it is defined and measurable.

Developing a Consistent Routine

A daily routine that incorporates activities related to manifesting one's goals can help maintain motivation. This routine may include time dedicated to visualization, meditation, reading inspiring material, or journal writing. The consistency of these practices reinforces commitment and helps keep the mind focused and motivated.

Surrounding Oneself with Positive Support

The social environment can have a significant impact on our motivation. Surrounding oneself with people who support our efforts, who share similar visions, or who are simply positive can infuse energy and inspiration. Participating in groups or communities that value personal growth and manifestation can also offer support and encouragement in times of doubt or frustration.

Use of Affirmations and Visualizations

Positive affirmations and visualization sessions, as extensively explained in the book, can be powerful tools for maintaining the right attitude and reinforcing internal motivation. Repeating affirmations that echo desired goals helps realign the subconscious mind towards these goals, while visualizing oneself as having already achieved those goals can enhance desire and action towards them.

Managing Expectations

Finally, it is essential to manage one's expectations. Being realistic about timing and possible obstacles can prevent disappointments and demotivation. Understanding that manifestation is a process that may take time helps maintain a balanced perspective and remain patient and persistent.

In summary, maintaining motivation requires a holistic approach that integrates practical methods and emotional support. Through celebrating progress, clarity of goals, community support, the use of self-development tools, and realistic expectation management, it is possible to navigate periods of stagnation with unaltered motivation, continuously guiding towards the realization of one's dreams.

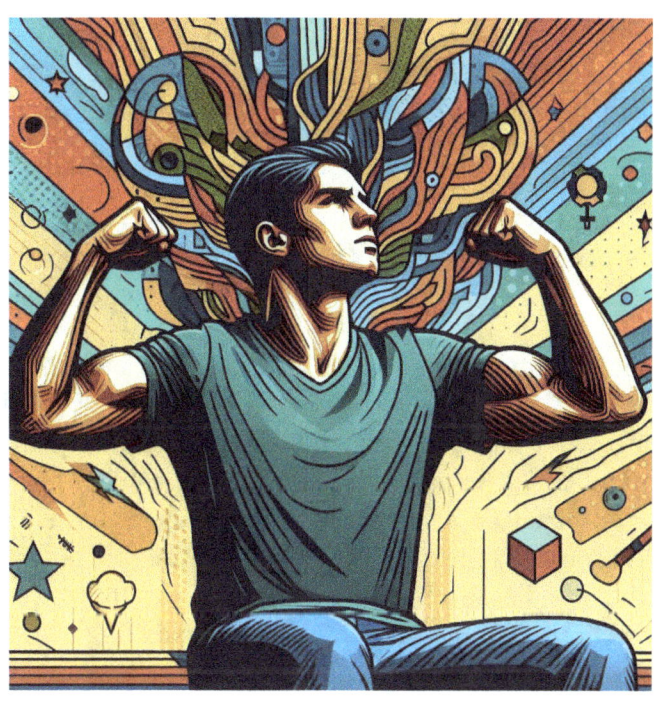

ADAPTABILITY AND RESILIENCE

In a rapidly changing world, adaptability and resilience have become essential skills, not only for navigating daily challenges but also for thriving in any context. Remaining flexible and responsive to changes can mean the difference between successfully overcoming obstacles and falling behind. This ability to adapt and quickly recover from difficulties is particularly critical in the manifestation process, where things often don't go according to the planned.

Understanding Adaptability and Resilience

Adaptability and resilience are two interconnected qualities that play a crucial role in individuals' ability to effectively navigate through life's changes and challenges. Adaptability, in particular, refers to the ability to change one's behavior and way of thinking in response to new environments, challenges, or conditions. This mental agility allows individuals to remain effective and functional in the face of change, adapting strategies, goals, and actions according to changing circumstances. Being adaptable means being flexible, open to the new, and ready to revise plans when necessary, without losing sight of long-term goals.

On the other hand, resilience is the ability to bounce back quickly from difficulties and adversity. It is a form of psychological toughness that allows people to "bounce back" after failures, disappointments, or periods of stress. Unlike adaptability, which is more oriented towards adaptation and modification, resilience focuses on the ability to regain strength and morale despite setbacks. This quality is crucial for maintaining a positive outlook on life, a sense of hope, and optimism even when things don't go as planned.

Both of these qualities are essential for anyone wishing to pursue personal and professional success in a rapidly changing world. Adaptability allows people to be versatile and inventive, capable of exploring new opportunities and finding creative solutions to problems. Similarly, resilience provides the inner strength needed to face challenges without becoming discouraged, promoting perseverance and the ability to overcome obstacles.

The interaction between adaptability and resilience creates a powerful dynamic that equips individuals not only to survive but to thrive. An adaptable individual can change tactics effortlessly and explore new paths, while their resilience enables them to face and overcome any difficulties that these new paths may present. Together, these qualities help navigate through uncertainty and change with a combination of strategic flexibility and emotional robustness, crucial for fully realizing one's potential in every aspect of life.

Developing Adaptability

1. **Growth Mindset**:

Adopting a growth mindset is essential for adaptability. This involves seeing challenges as opportunities to learn and grow rather than insurmountable obstacles. Those who possess a growth mindset are more inclined to experiment with new solutions and approaches, facilitating adaptation in unexpected situations.

2. **Intentional Exposure to New Experiences:**

Regularly exposing oneself to new situations can improve adaptability. This can include traveling, learning new skills, or simply changing the daily routine. Each new experience builds the repertoire of responses that a person can use when facing changes.

3. **Continuous Feedback:**

Being open to feedback and using it to make adjustments is vital. Feedback, whether from colleagues, friends, or mentors, can provide valuable insights into how one is adapting and which areas require improvement.

Cultivating Resilience

1. **Support Network**:

Having a solid support network is crucial for resilience. Support from family, friends, or colleagues can provide not only comfort and advice during periods of stress but also practical resources that can help overcome challenges.

2. **Self-Care Practices**:

Maintaining regular self-care practices improves overall resilience to stress. This includes activities such as physical exercise, meditation, relaxing hobbies, or adequate rest. Self-care not only strengthens physical health but also stabilizes emotional balance, making individuals less vulnerable to external pressures.

3. **Planning and Preparation**:

Being prepared for potential setbacks can increase resilience. This may mean having backup plans, reserve resources, or emergency strategies ready to be implemented when needed. Preparing for the worst while hoping for the best is a pragmatic approach that can reduce anxiety and increase confidence in one's ability to handle challenges.

Conclusions

In conclusion, adaptability and resilience are not only desirable traits but essential for anyone aspiring to a satisfying and productive life in an ever-changing context. Developing these skills means enhancing one's ability to navigate uncertainties and changes with confidence and determination, ensuring not only survival but thriving in every aspect of life.

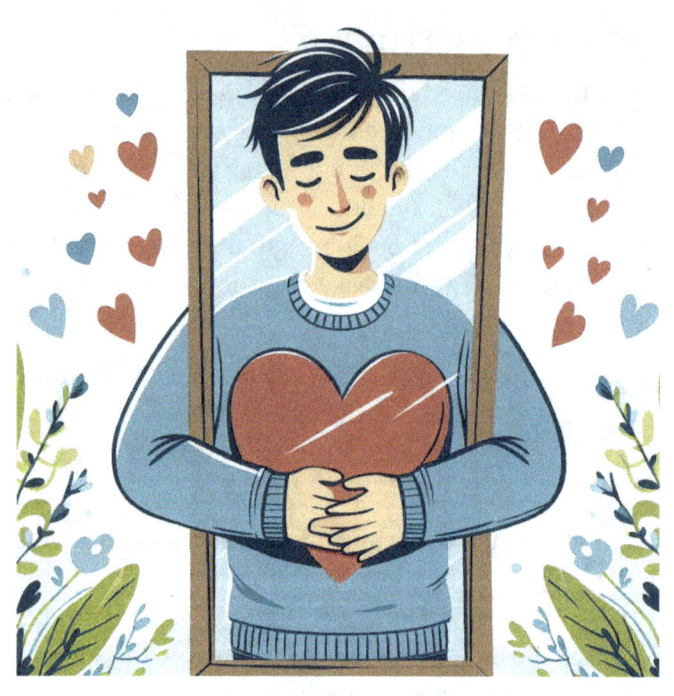

CONCLUSION

SUMMARY OF KEY POINTS
SYNTHESIS OF THE MOST IMPORTANT
TECHNIQUES AND CONCEPTS

Conclusion

Through this journey of exploration and understanding of the techniques and fundamental principles of manifestation, we have examined a variety of strategies and key concepts that are essential for anyone wishing to transform their dreams and goals into tangible realities. Here is a summary of the most important points we have discussed, serving as a concluding synthesis and as a guide for your personal manifestation practice.

Clarity of Goals

One of the fundamental pillars of manifestation is the clarity of goals. Having well-defined, specific, and measurable goals not only provides clear direction but also facilitates progress monitoring and helps maintain motivation along the way. The application of the SMART methodology (Specific, Measurable, Achievable, Relevant, Time-bound) has been emphasized as an effective approach to structuring goals that are not only clear but also achievable.

Maintaining Motivation

We have explored various strategies for maintaining motivation, particularly important in times when results are slow to manifest. Celebrating small successes, setting intermediate milestones, and developing a daily routine that incorporates manifestation practices are all elements that contribute to sustained commitment. Additionally, surrounding oneself with positive support, both through relationships and inspirational environments, is crucial for nurturing continuous enthusiasm towards one's goals.

Adaptability and Resilience

The ability to adapt to changes and resilience in the face of obstacles are crucial qualities in the manifestation process. Adaptability allows navigating uncertainties with flexibility and creativity, while resilience provides the strength to overcome challenges and continue pursuing goals despite difficulties. These qualities not only help overcome obstacles but also transform challenges into opportunities for growth and learning.

Visualization and Affirmation Techniques

Visualization techniques and positive affirmations are powerful tools that reinforce intention and facilitate manifestation. Visualization helps create a clear mental image of the desired outcome, while affirmations serve to mentally strengthen belief and positive expectation. Both of these practices are essential for aligning the subconscious with conscious goals and attracting desired circumstances.

Continued Support and Lifelong Learning

Finally, ongoing support and lifelong learning have emerged as vital elements for long-term success in manifestation. Access to educational resources, participation in support groups, and continuous seeking of feedback are practices that contribute to a continuous deepening of manifestation techniques and a better understanding of oneself.

In conclusion, while the journey towards realizing one's desires may be complex and challenging, the techniques and concepts explored offer a solid and proven framework for effectively guiding your aspirations towards manifestation. By remembering and applying these principles, you will be better equipped to navigate the journey of manifestation with confidence, determination, and, above all, success.

CALL TO ACTION

ENCOURAGEMENT TO YOU, READERS, TO BEGIN YOUR MANIFESTATION JOURNEY

Now that we have explored together the techniques, strategies, and essential principles of manifestation, the next step is yours. It's time to move from theory to practice, to put into action the knowledge you have acquired, and to start your personal journey towards realizing your dreams and goals. Here's a clear invitation to take courage and take that bold first step towards manifesting your desired reality.

1. **Define Your Goals**: Take a moment to reflect on your deepest aspirations. What are the dreams you want to turn into reality? Be clear and specific in your goals, use the SMART methodology to formulate them effectively, and write everything down on paper.

2. **Commit to a Daily Routine**: Establish a daily routine that includes visualization practices, positive affirmations, and moments of reflection. Make these practices a non-negotiable part of your day, just as you would for any other activity important for your health or well-being.

3. **Surround Yourself with Positivity**: Be selective about the people you spend time with and the environments you find yourself in. Surround yourself with support and inspiration, whether through nurturing

friendships, support groups, or simply consuming media that reinforces your vision and motivation.

4. **Monitor and Celebrate Your Progress**: Keep track of your progress and take the time to celebrate every small success along the way. This will not only keep your motivation high but also help you see how far you've already come.

5. **Adapt and Persist:** Be ready to make adjustments along the way. Manifestation is a dynamic process, and flexibility is your ally. If you encounter obstacles, use your resilience to find solutions and keep pushing forward with renewed vigor.

Don't let your aspirations remain confined to dreams, hidden among thoughts of what "could be" or "might have been." Every great journey begins with a single, determined step, and yours begins right here and now, in this moment full of unexplored potential. Always remember that the ability to manifest your reality is firmly in your hands; you are the architect and creator of your destiny. Start shaping your world with intention, with constant commitment, and with unwavering faith in your intrinsic capabilities.

This moment is not just a mere interval in the flow of time but a clear and powerful signal to begin. It's an invitation to take the reins of your life and steer the narrative towards outcomes of success and fulfillment. Let your manifestation journey unfold in all its magnificent transformative potential. With every small daily action, with every decision made consciously, and with every intentional step towards your goals, you are building the structure of the life you want to live.

Now, ask yourself: what action can I take today to bring myself even one step closer to my dreams? No matter how small this step may seem, every forward movement is vital. The time to act is now. Not tomorrow, not next week, but today. The urgency to live the life you desire should be palpable, pushing you to act with courage and determination.

This is your time. This is your call to action. Be bold, be resilient, and above all, be committed to the path you have chosen. The road to manifestation is both bright and challenging, but with every conscious step, you will come closer to realizing your boldest dreams. And in doing so, you will discover not only the power to fulfill your desires but also the depth of your inner strength and capacity for transformation. So, move, act, and start turning the possible into reality.

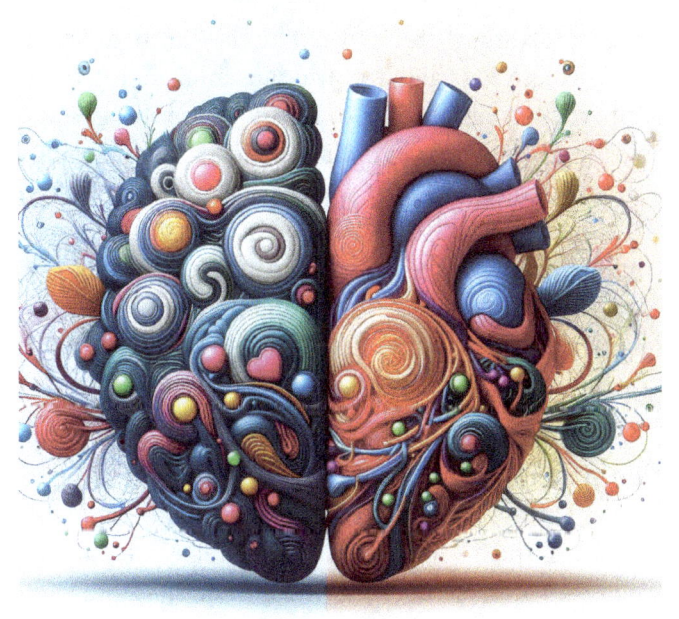

FINAL REFLECTIONS: DRAWING FROM THE WISDOM OF DOLORES CANNON

Closure with Motivational Thoughts on the Power of One's Mind

As we approach the conclusion of this journey of exploration and growth, it becomes essential to reflect on the extraordinary influence that the mind exerts on our existence, a recurring and fundamental theme in Dolores Cannon's teachings. Her thorough research and practices developed over the years have clearly demonstrated to us how the reality in which we live is significantly shaped by our thoughts and beliefs. Dolores Cannon has repeatedly emphasized that the human mind goes far beyond the passive role of a mere instrument for interpreting the surrounding reality; rather, it is a powerful creative agent capable of shaping and transforming the world in which we live.

This understanding leads us to recognize the immense responsibility we have in managing our thoughts and beliefs. If the mind can create reality, then it becomes crucial to consciously nurture thoughts that not only reflect our true desires and highest aspirations but also promote an enriching and positive existence. The implications of this principle are vast: every thought, every fragment of belief we nurture, contributes to weaving the fabric of our daily lives. Dolores Cannon has taught us that, with the right awareness and attention, we can direct and shape this creative capacity of the mind to improve not only our personal lives but also positively influence the world around us. This requires an active commitment to maintaining a steady flow of positive and constructive thoughts, challenging negative or limiting mental habits we may have developed.

Dolores Cannon's approach, therefore, invites us to consider the mind as a tool for personal and collective transformation, a source of creative power that, when well directed, can lead to significant and lasting changes. With this new understanding, we are called to act with a renewed awareness of our potential, recognizing that every moment of thought is an opportunity to build and enrich our reality. This final reflection aims to motivate you to exercise this power with wisdom and intention, to actively transform your life and, cascadingly, the world around you.

Dolores Cannon has frequently explored and discussed the concept of the "superconscious mind," emphasizing its crucial role not only in our spiritual development but also in our material existence. According to Cannon, accessing this elevated part of our consciousness opens the doors to levels of knowledge and understanding that far exceed our daily experience. This access not only allows us to discover hidden aspects of our being but also equips us with powerful tools to co-create and actively influence our reality. This view reminds us that we are much more complex and profound beings than our daily experiences and physical bodies may suggest.

Incorporating these profound reflections, it becomes essential to adopt a perspective on thoughts that sees them not as mere ephemeral products of our brain but as true seeds of potentiality. If these seeds are cultivated with intent and awareness, they have the potential to blossom into concrete and tangible results. Every decision we make, every reaction we show, and every thought we nurture actively shapes the structure and fabric of our lives. Thoughts, however transient or insignificant they may seem, are in reality immensely powerful and laden with creative potential.

Dolores Cannon has taught us that every thought we nurture is meaningful; each one contributes to shaping our path and our destiny. Through awareness and attention, we can learn to consciously direct these thoughts towards the goals and realities we wish to manifest. This process of intentional direction is not only an act of personal creation but becomes a journey of transformation that can profoundly alter our way of living and interacting with the world.

This understanding invites us to assess every thought, every moment of awareness as a precious opportunity to actively build the desired reality. The superconscious mind, therefore, is not just a detached or inaccessible part of us; it is a living source of creative potential that, once fully embraced and utilized, can lead us to destinies we once could only imagine. With this approach, we commit not only to living in the world but to shaping it, guided by the profound wisdom that Dolores Cannon has shared with us.

Therefore, remember to exercise your power with wisdom and awareness. Your mind is not just a factory of thoughts but a powerful transmitter of energy that deeply influences yourself and the surrounding environment. Dolores Cannon has strongly emphasized how our inner energy, when directed positively, can catalyze processes of healing, growth, and radical transformation. This principle is not limited solely to our personal lives; it also extends to the lives of those around us, influencing communities and shared spaces through the vibrations we emit.

This power requires great responsibility—being aware that every thought, every emotion, and every action sends ripples into the fabric of reality, altering it in visible and invisible ways. Dolores Cannon has taught us that we can use this ability to trigger positive change, not only for ourselves but also for the world around us, highlighting that personal healing is often the first step towards collective healing.

As you proceed on your manifestation journey, treasure the words and teachings of Dolores Cannon. Let the awareness of the extraordinary power of your mind guide and inspire you every day. Be bold in your aspirations, mindful and determined in your actions, and always remain open to the infinite possibilities that your mind can accomplish. Every thought you nurture is a seed that, if cultivated with care, can grow and bloom into tangible realities that enrich your life and the lives of others.

This is the time to fully embrace your creative power and to begin living the life you have always dreamed of. The journey is yours to explore and define. Take this moment as a sign to begin, an invitation to move with confidence and joy towards the future you desire. Let your manifestation journey unfold in all its wonderful and transformative potentialities. This is not just a possibility; it is a call to action, an appeal to live fully, harnessing the extraordinary capacity of your mind to shape reality. Venture forth with courage and discover how deep and fulfilling the journey can be when guided by the knowledge and inspiration that Dolores Cannon has left as a legacy.

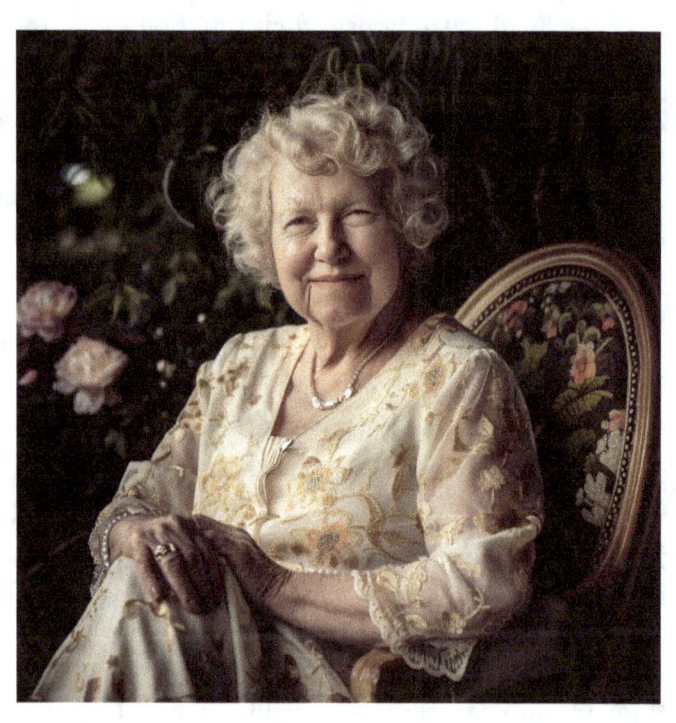

APPENDIX: ADDITIONAL RESOURCES

As you continue your journey of personal and spiritual growth, it's essential to have access to resources that can provide insights, techniques, and inspiration. Understanding and practicing manifestation, as taught by Dolores Cannon and other experts in the field, can be enriched and deepened through a variety of materials and learning opportunities. Below, you'll find a curated selection of books, articles, workshops, and courses that will help you expand your knowledge and refine your practice.

Books

1. **"The Convoluted Universe"** series by Dolores Cannon - This series of books offers a deep dive into Cannon's discoveries through her practice of past life regression. Each volume explores complex concepts of existence and consciousness in ways that challenge and expand traditional perceptions of reality.

2. **"The Power of Now"** by Eckhart Tolle - A classic on spirituality and mind control, this book is essential for anyone wishing to better understand the power of living in the present and its relationship to manifesting desires.

3. **"Ask and It Is Given"** by Esther and Jerry Hicks (The Teachings of Abraham) - This book introduces readers to the law of attraction, offering practical exercises to improve the ability to attract what you want

in life.

Articles

1. **"Harnessing the Power of the Mind for Healing and Manifestation"** - Available on various scientific publication platforms, this article explores the intersections between mind, body, and healing, emphasizing how thoughts influence physical reality.

2. **"The Science Behind Manifestation"** - This article, available in online magazines like Psychology Today, analyzes studies and psychological theories supporting the manifestation process, providing a scientific perspective on how and why it works.

Workshops and Courses

1. Quantum Healing Hypnosis Technique (QHHT) Certification - For those seriously interested in following in Dolores Cannon's footsteps, QHHT certification courses offer comprehensive training on conducting hypnosis sessions for past life regression, teaching techniques for accessing the superconscious mind.

2. Manifestation Workshops - Many spirituality experts and life coaches offer workshops both online and in-person, where participants can learn advanced techniques to hone their manifestation abilities. These workshops often include guided visualization sessions, intention-setting exercises, and strategies for overcoming mental blocks.

3. Online Courses on Spiritual Growth and Personal Development - Platforms like Udemy, Coursera, and MasterClass offer courses covering a wide range of topics, from personal development to spiritual growth, all useful for those wishing to deepen their self-improvement and manifestation journey.

Using these resources can greatly enhance your understanding and ability to effectively apply manifestation techniques in your life. Each book, article, and course is a step toward greater self-mastery and understanding of the world around you, allowing you to live with greater intentionality and fulfill your deepest dreams.

Practical Exercises: Supplementary Activities for the Reader

To further enrich your manifestation journey and help you integrate the lessons learned, here you will find a selection of additional practical exercises. These exercises are designed to stimulate reflection, enhance your manifestation abilities, and help you directly experience the influence of your thoughts and actions on the reality around you.

1. **Vision Board**

   - **Objective**: Clearly visualize your desires and aspirations.

   - **How to do it**: Take a large sheet of paper and draw a

map connecting your main goals with the specific steps needed to achieve them. Use images, words, symbols, or collages that represent your dreams. This visual map will serve as a daily reminder of your aspirations and the path you intend to follow to achieve them.

2. Gratitude Journal

- **Objective**: Cultivate an attitude of gratitude, which is essential for attracting abundance and positivity.

- **How to do it**: Every evening, before going to sleep, write down three things you are grateful for that day. This exercise helps you focus your attention on the positive, increasing your energetic frequency and enhancing your ability to attract what you desire.

3. Personalized Affirmations

- **Objective**: Strengthen your self-efficacy and confidence in your manifestation abilities.

- **How to do it**: Write a series of positive affirmations that reflect your goals and the qualities you want to attract or reinforce in yourself. Examples of affirmations could be: "I am a powerful creator of my reality" or "I easily welcome abundance and success into my life." Repeat these affirmations every morning and evening, and whenever you feel the need for reinforcement.

4. Visualization Meditation

- **Objective**: Strengthen the connection with your goals by clearly visualizing them.

- **How to do it**: Dedicate 10-15 minutes each day to meditation, focusing on visualizing your goals as if they have already been achieved. Feel the emotions, observe the details, and experience the situation as if it were real in that moment. This practice not only improves your mood but also strengthens your manifestation ability.

5. **Barrier Analysis**

   - **Objective**: Identify and overcome internal obstacles hindering manifestation.

   - **How to do it**: Write a list of fears or limiting beliefs that you feel may be holding back your success. Next to each point, write a countermeasure or action you can take to overcome these barriers. This exercise helps you become more aware of your internal blocks and actively work to resolve them.

These practical exercises are powerful tools for developing and deepening your manifestation practice. By integrating these activities into your daily routine, you can not only improve your understanding and application of manifestation techniques but also accelerate your progress toward realizing your deepest desires.

GLOSSARY

In this glossary, you will find a collection of terms and key concepts used in the book. This summary will help you better understand the principles of manifestation and deepen your study and personal practice.

1. **Manifestation**: The process through which thoughts, intentions, and beliefs translate into tangible reality. It is the act of bringing into physical reality what was previously imagined or desired at the mental level.

2. **Supraconscious Mind**: Term used by Dolores Cannon to describe a higher part of the human consciousness that transcends ordinary awareness and allows access to higher knowledge and powers, including the ability to influence and alter material reality.

3. **Law of Attraction**: Metaphysical principle stating that similar energy attracts similar energy. In the practice of manifestation, it refers to the concept that positive thoughts and emotions attract positive events and circumstances into a person's life.

4. **Visualization**: Meditation or reflection technique involving the mental creation of vivid and detailed images of desired scenarios. It is used to enhance focus and intention in manifesting one's goals.

5. **Affirmations**: Positive and repeated statements aimed at strengthening confidence in personal abilities and promoting positive changes in a person's life. Affirmations are used to restructure thinking and fuel personal transformation.

6. **Resilience**: The ability to quickly recover from difficulties; the ability to bounce back after adversity or failure while maintaining a positive outlook despite challenges.

7. **Adaptability**: The ability to modify one's behavior and thinking in response to new environments, challenges, or conditions; a form of mental agility that enables individuals to remain effective in the face of change.

8. **QHHT (Quantum Healing Hypnosis Technique)**: Hypnosis technique developed by Dolores Cannon that facilitates access to the supraconscious mind for healing and spiritual exploration purposes, through past life regression and communication with the Higher Self.

9. **Inner Energy**: Refers to a person's life force or psychic energy, which can be directed or shaped through mindfulness and intention practices to influence physical reality.

10. **Intention**: The motivational force behind an

individual's actions; in the context of manifestation, it refers to the clear and deliberate direction of thought and energy towards the realization of specific goals.

These terms form the foundations of manifestation techniques and provide guidance for their practical and theoretical use. By deepening your understanding of these concepts, you can more effectively apply manifestation techniques in your daily life and move closer to realizing your desires.

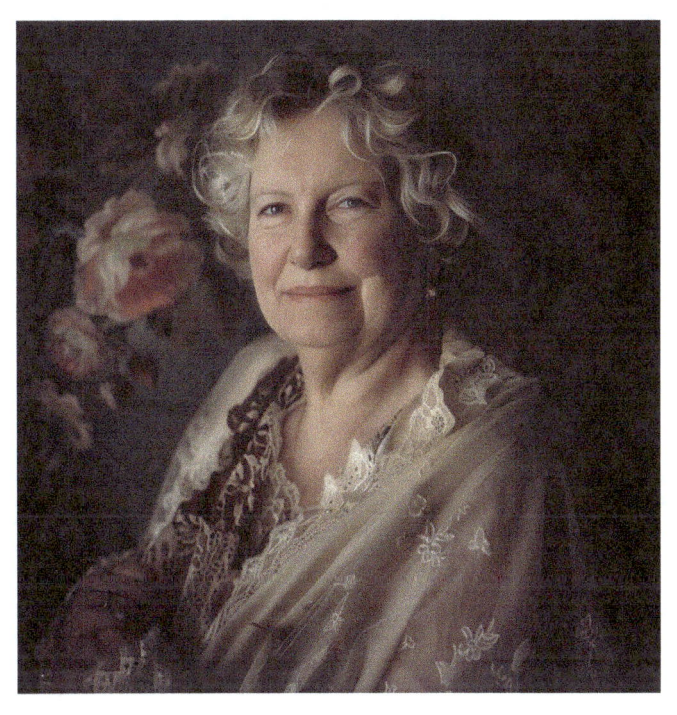

www.ingramcontent.com/pod-product-compliance
Lightning Source LLC
Chambersburg PA
CBHW052254220526
45471CB00001B/337